FITNESS
WITHOUT FAIL

Vine Hill Publishing

FITNESS
WITHOUT FAIL

How To Stick With ANY
Exercise Routine

**THE LITTLE-KNOWN SECRETS FOR
STAYING TRUE TO YOUR FITNESS GOALS**

BILL R. JUDSON

ISBN: 978-0-9976168-5-9

Cover and interior design by Ngirl Design

Proofreading by Last Word Proofreading

Vine Hill Publishing
P.O. Box 308
Forestville, CA 95436

Printed in the United States of America

Library of Congress Control Number: 2016908322

First Edition

*In memory of my mother, Connie,
whose love for books and love for
me made this book possible.*

*Also to my son, Lance, for the joy
he has brought to my life.*

Acknowledgements

This book would not have been possible without so many people sharing both their fitness struggles and victories with me. Thank you to all who have shared your stories and experiences.

My editors, Catherine Adams of Inkslinger and Robin Bethel of Prose Studio, deserve much credit in smoothing the rough edges of my material, to put it mildly. They were a sheer pleasure to work with and amazingly inspirational.

I'm also thankful to Steve Harrison and Jack Canfield for the knowledge and advice they have shared with me. The education and wisdom they provided made the job of producing this book much easier.

And finally, a heartfelt thanks to my brothers and sisters for their unwavering confidence in me.

Contents

Introduction

Sticking with an exercise routine is difficult. You and everyone else have found this out. A structure that would dwarf the Eiffel Tower could be built from all the exercise equipment that is now just a place to hang clothes. If the money from unused gym memberships filled your pockets each month, you'd be a billionaire before the year was through.

Still, we all know some diehards who are able to pull it off. How do they *do it*? This book will answer an even more important question: How can *you* do it?

This book will help put an end to the struggle. You'll learn how to stay engaged with fitness and keep your fitness program from suddenly evaporating. Imagine being able to get in shape and stay that way. With this book you can make that a reality.

Engaging in sufficient exercise has become a worldwide problem. The Harvard School of Public Health reports, "Globally, about one in three people gets little, if any, physical activity." Studies of activity levels in the U.S. are consistent with this global trend. The 2012 survey conducted by the National Center for Health Statistics found that "According to the 2008 federal physical activity guidelines for aerobic activity, 30% of adults were inactive, 20% of adults were insufficiently active, and 50% were sufficiently active based on their participation in leisure-time physical activity."

While this represents a slight improvement over their survey results from previous years, the troubling fact remains that about half of adults still do not get enough exercise—in spite of having more available facilities, programs, and personal trainers than ever before. It's also in spite of continuous messaging from multiple sources promoting all the reasons we should exercise.

So why are many of us still inactive? One major reason is that while we have more opportunities and incentives to exercise, we have little information on how to motivate ourselves to actually do it. For years, I searched for a practical guide I could give people that would help them stick with exercise. I never quite found it. Eventually, I realized that if I was serious about helping others, I needed to take it upon myself to create such a guide.

To create this book, I observed what separates those who exercise regularly from those who don't. I noticed what works for me, listened to what works for those around me, read what industry experts had to say, and studied the latest fitness research. I also sought wisdom from masters in the fields of motivation, personal development, and human psychology.

For a long time I had nothing but a massive collection of seemingly unrelated bits of data, advice, tips, and philosophies. It was like trying to put together a 1,000 piece puzzle using a handful of pieces from many different boxes. Some of the pieces fit together, but not nearly enough to create a clear picture. Clouding the matter even further was how people are so different. What brings joy to one person may bring misery to another.

I was beginning to see why no one had yet developed a cohesive guide that anyone could use. It just didn't seem possible. Still, my desire to help people live healthier, happier lives wouldn't allow me to stop until I had somehow found a way.

At long last, subtle patterns began to emerge from my research. While everybody is, in fact, unique, there is a deeper level at which we're all the same. Regardless of our age, gender, or life circumstances, we're all human with human tendencies, such as preferring pleasure over pain and acting according to how we see ourselves. When I rearranged the puzzle pieces according to basic human traits, I found the clear picture I had been searching for.

What I discovered is that it all comes down to inspiring our human nature to work for us rather than against us. Just as we can count on water to run downhill, there are certain human traits we can count on. Using these to our advantage lies at the heart of transforming exercise from a struggle into a treasured part of our day. Fighting against ourselves doesn't work. The key is to make human nature our friend rather than our foe.

You'll find this book different from many other fitness books in that it doesn't prescribe a particular fitness program or routine. One-size-fits-all programs are inherently short-term solutions. Exercise programs need to be as unique and individual as the people undertaking them. What you decide to do and how you decide to do it need to be highly personalized for long-term success. In this book, you'll discover how to leverage your natural human nature to create a personal approach to fitness that aligns with who you are. And when exercise becomes an extension of the person you are, you'll find that it earns a place in your life for a lifetime.

This book offers a comprehensive, cohesive approach that touches on all of the mental, physical, and emotional facets of a fitness program. Concepts are presented in an order designed to maximize their effect. The teachings, however, aren't interdependent; each of the concepts holds independent power and ability to help us, which means that you'll start to benefit almost right away. By the end of Chapter 2, you'll already have tools you can use to make it easier to stay consistent with exercise. Success is not dependent on strict application of every point. It's quite possible only one of them is the missing ingredient that you need.

A gradual progression into an active lifestyle is recommended within this book for multiple reasons, not the least of which is your safety. Moderate increases in activity level are safe for most people, but those with risk factors for certain diseases like diabetes or cardiovascular disease should consult with their doctor at the outset of increasing activity levels.

It's my sincere hope you'll take advantage of the teachings you find within these pages to become the fit and vibrant person you'd like to be. If you would like more information and support beyond this book, I invite you to visit my website at www.fitnesswithoutfail.com.

Bill R. Judson

PART I

Leveraging Human Nature

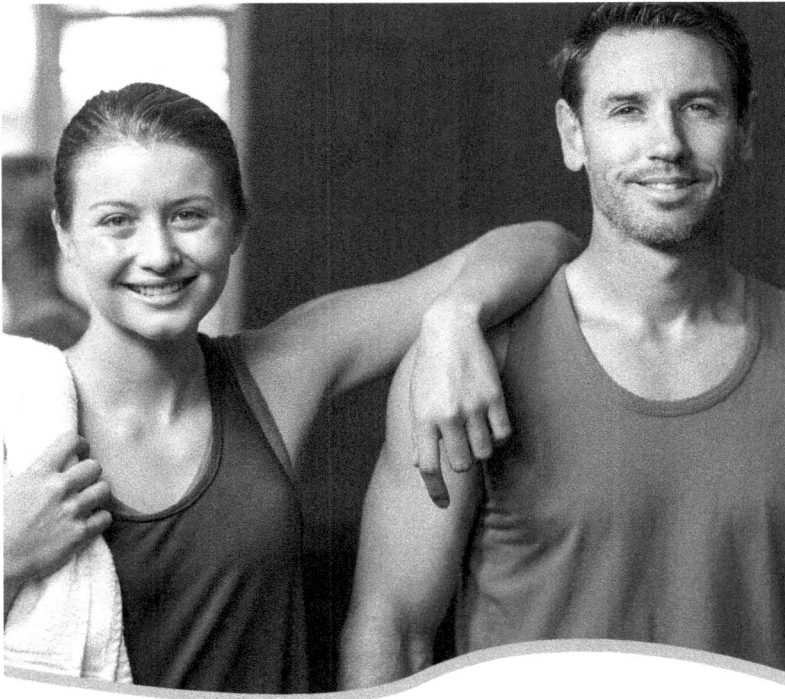

Part I focuses on how to orient yourself mentally, emotionally, and socially in order to make exercise a regular and enduring part of your life. You breed success by aligning exercise, your inner world, and natural tendencies.

Chapter 1

A New Approach

"Look deep into nature, and then
you will understand everything better."

Albert Einstein

Success Rates

Every morning Karen opened her closet door with a deep sigh and began rifling through her clothes, trying to find something that would still fit. Her frustration grew daily until she reached a tipping point. She couldn't continue down this path; she had to do something about it. Rather than buying larger clothes again, Karen set a New Year's resolution: *this year* she was going to exercise every week. She would finally get her money's worth from that gym membership she'd been paying for but not using.

Karen started off pretty well. The first week she made it to the gym three times—and even four times the next week. It wasn't easy, but she was determined. In the third week things got hectic and she only made it twice. She scolded herself sufficiently to rebound back to three workouts the following week. But again, she slipped to two workouts in the next week, and one in the next, until she stopped going altogether. She had lots of reasons why she stopped going. None of them were the real reason.

Karen's story is all too familiar to many of us. We start exercising with the best of intentions, but it's not long before our initial zeal fades and we find ourselves as inactive as before. Studies monitoring the dropout rates for people who start a new exercise program have found about half will quit within the first six months, with the majority of dropouts occurring during the first 12 weeks. Fitness clubs typically have a substantial percentage of members who attend less than once a week and 90% of clubs will lose 30% to 50% of its members each year.

These statistics are reflected in our own lives and social circles. Think of all the people you know. How many of them exercise regularly? What percentage would you estimate? Most of us know a few people that exercise regularly, but they're usually far outnumbered by those who don't.

What You Need to Know

While it's normal to have difficulty staying fit, this doesn't have to be your fate. You're about to discover why most struggle and why you no longer have to.

Not exercising when we know we should while also seeing that some people *are* successful in exercising regularly draws us to conclude we are somehow deficient. We come to believe that we must not have the same willpower others do or we weren't born with the yet undiscovered exercise gene they've been blessed with.

But this isn't the case. Karen, from our story, isn't lazy, weak, or in possession of some other character flaw. It's simply a matter of what she doesn't know.

So what is it that those who exercise regularly know or do differently from the rest? This is where it gets complicated. There isn't a common approach everyone uses. Question several people about how they stay consistent with exercise and you'll get many different answers.

The Common Thread

Growing up, I discovered I had a talent. I could eat an insane amount of food in one sitting. I could eat more than anyone I knew. It was fun to amaze people by putting away copious quantities of food. Having witnessed my ability on so many occasions, my friends confidently challenged anyone that boasted they were capable of mass consumption to duel me at the table.

By the time I got into college and was no longer competing in sports, this talent started to show its consequence and I started to gain weight. It was plain to see that once I graduated from college and secured a desk job, the combination of my eating habits and hours of sitting would lead me to become too large to fit through doorways. I decided I needed to start exercising, but multiple attempts all failed miserably.

After college, I tried a different approach to exercise. Thankfully, I had more success this time. As time went on, there were things I did somewhat incidentally that further integrated exercise into my identity and lifestyle. What was the secret to my success in exercising consistently through all of the many (many, many) years since college? Luck. I was lucky enough to pick an approach that fit my particular personality and stumbled into doing other things that reinforced it.

The one common denominator of people who exercise consistently has typically been that they were able to develop fitness as a fixture in their lives without having been told how. It didn't happen because of something they were born with or that someone taught them. Gradually, over time, they managed to figure out what works for them.

Learning something through trial and error without the benefit of coaching is always a long process. Most people become discouraged and quit before gaining enough experience. They don't know what they should do . . . and why should they?

It pains me to see how many people feel like failures because they haven't been able to stick with an exercise program. It's as though we expect it to be instinctual and not something we need to be taught. The truth is it's a learned skill that nobody teaches us (but should).

Would we expect a child to develop good manners if they were never taught? Did we expect to learn to drive a car without someone showing us how? These are much less difficult skills than maintaining a consistent exercise regime, yet we fully expect them to be taught.

Where in your upbringing or schooling were you taught the things that make it easier to stick with an exercise routine? Were you taught in school by your physical education teacher? Did your parents tell you or show you by example? Is there an adult education class you could have taken? Is there some person or organization that offered to give you this information?

It's not that people have been holding out on you. None of the people around you really knew, either. No one taught them. If you've been lucky, you know some people who have figured a few things out for themselves and shared those tips with you. Chances are, though, you've had very little, if any, help.

Our Changing World

Knowledge on how to develop the skills we need to maintain an active lifestyle is limited because we've only recently developed a need for those skills. In relatively recent history, most people's lives required plenty of exercise just to survive. Staying warm and cooking food required gathering and chopping wood. Water had to be fetched. Food had to be hunted or grown. Imagine the workout you would get washing clothes using a washboard. Almost anything a person wanted required doing something physical in order to have it. There was no need to teach people how to stay active.

At first gradually and now rapidly, our daily existence has come to require less and less physical activity. Technology and other advancements have replaced the need for us to move our bodies. It was not long ago that if you wanted to buy something, you at least needed to get up, walk to your car, drive to the store, park, walk into the store, walk through aisles browsing for your items, stand in line at the checkout, pack your purchases into your car, drive home, and carry what you bought into your house. All this activity can now be replaced with a little wiggling of your fingers as we simply buy online. We think it's great that we saved all that time and effort. The problem is our body needed that effort.

Physical activity is no longer an inherent part of the American lifestyle. The never-ending stream of new devices and technologies has brought us to the point where movement has become optional. From 1950 to 2000, the percentage of the U.S. population working in low-activity jobs nearly doubled. From 1960 to 2000, the percentage of trips to work using automobiles rose from 67% to 88%. From 1969 to 2001, the percentage of children who walked or rode a bicycle to school dropped from 40% to 13%. The average American now spends 88% of their time sitting. These types of changes are not unique to the U.S. There is a worldwide decline in physical activity.

> "The end of the human race will be that it eventually dies of civilization."
> **Ralph Waldo Emerson**

These days, a person could easily get a job working from home and have everything that is needed or wanted delivered right to the door. All entertainment and social contact could be streamed through the Internet. He or she could live a life very close to "normal" by today's standards with almost no movement whatsoever.

Our bodies are designed to hunt, gather, and travel great distances by foot. They don't function well when they're not used. Species evolve and adapt, of course, but the process takes thousands of years. Our bodies haven't had nearly enough time to adapt to being used so little.

> "It is impossible to overlook the extent civilization is built upon a renunciation of instinct."
>
> **Sigmund Freud**

Our DNA still includes a primal need for movement. We were connected to it as babies and children, but with each passing year our parents and society enforced increasing limits on our behavior, until this part of us was eventually subdued. Our culture has largely domesticated our instinct to move, leaving us out of sync with our nature.

This disparity between what our bodies are engineered for and how we actually use them has created a host of problems. The increased incident of diseases like heart disease, obesity, and diabetes is alarming. This incongruence also manifests itself in many other ways, including decreased energy and vitality. By discouraging movement, society diminishes our ability to achieve optimum health and happiness. Good health isn't merely the absence of disease. At the core, human beings are complex, integrated energy systems and a lack of adequate body movement impedes these systems. Our mind, body, and spirit are interconnected. When we neglect to honor the body with the activity it needs, our mind and spirit suffer, too.

The Void

Since our lives no longer force us to move, we must be taught. We need to be taught how much movement the body needs and how to make that movement a normal and natural part of our lives.

There are an infinite number of exercise programs you could follow. Bookstores are loaded with books and magazines that provide "how to" advice for a wide variety of activities. Want to run a marathon? Pump iron? Follow an A-list program endorsed by movie stars? The book is waiting. There is no shortage of advice on how to become fit.

But what you *won't* find is sufficient guidance on how to get yourself to do any of it. This is what you need above anything else, isn't it? A lack of activity coaching is not what holds us back. You already know how to walk, jog, and ride a bicycle, and fitness classes provide instruction once you're there. The problem is rather how to get yourself off the couch and out the door.

The best fitness program in the world is useless if you can't get yourself to follow it. Knowing how to get yourself to the gym is more important than knowing what you'll do once you arrive. Naturally, it's also important to know what you're doing, and I'll take you through some helpful basics in later chapters. The essential starting point, though, is learning how to show up. Studying the rules of the road is a waste of time if we never sit behind the wheel.

With the lack of available instruction on how to incorporate consistent exercise into their lives, people have had to rely on random tips they've come across. These are often used in an attempt to build a relationship with exercise as one would with a boss. We have no choice but to work with our boss, so we try to get along as best we can. Even if we basically like our boss, our relationship is typically constrained by a sense of duty or obligation.

With this approach, exercise becomes just another job, an unrelenting boss making daily demands upon us. We eventually quit this job, because who needs another taskmaster?

Others assume it's simply a matter of mustering sufficient willpower to force ourselves to exercise. Nothing could be further from the truth. Trying to force yourself to do something you don't feel like doing won't work for long. An approach based primarily on self-discipline is guaranteed to eventually fail.

Your Success Formula

It's not surprising people tend to oversimplify what it takes to develop an exercise habit. The advice we've heard most often is "just do it." This advice for exercise is like learning to bake a soufflé with a recipe that simply says "turn on the oven." How many attempts would it take to guess the correct ingredients, mixture, time, and temperature? Cooking up a successful approach to staying fit is far more complex than baking a soufflé and requires a good recipe.

This book is designed to provide you with the recipe you need. Because exercise involves your whole being, the ingredients include physical, emotional, and psychological aspects. You'll gain the education, tools, and focus needed to successfully blend these ingredients to create and maintain a long-term fitness program. The most important thing you'll learn is how to take advantage of your human nature. Long-term success is found in cooperating with the natural world, rather than trying to fight against it.

The new approach you develop using this book will fit the unique person you are. You'll transform exercise from a dreary obligation into a cherished part of your day. Exercise will become a part of you and your identity in a way it never has been. And as it develops into an extension of the person you are, you'll find the health, fitness, and vitality you've longed for become a reality.

In the next chapter, we'll jump right into the specific steps you can take to build or improve your exercise habit. They are easy to follow and can create an immediate positive impact. To start building the tools that will transform your life, simply complete the action steps at the end of each of the following chapters.

CHAPTER HIGHLIGHTS

Success Rates
- The majority of people struggle to exercise consistently.

What You Need to Know
- Exercising regularly is a learned skill.

Your Success Formula
- Success is found through leveraging human nature.

Chapter 2

Get Going!

"Well begun is half done."

Aristotle

PREP to Exercise

In the previous chapter, I stated that maintaining fitness in the long run isn't primarily the result of dogged self-discipline. You're probably wondering, if this isn't the answer, then how is it achieved? This chapter begins to answer that question by first addressing what must happen before you'll do a workout.

There are four conditions that help enable exercise. It's not necessary to have all four for any given workout; in fact, having all four conditions present at once is rare. Even one of the four conditions is helpful, but the likelihood you'll do a workout increases as the conditions increase. If you have all four going for you, the workout is virtually guaranteed. The four conditions are:

1. **P**leasure
2. **R**outine
3. **E**nergy
4. **P**eople

When you want to exercise, remember you need to PREP first. Identify which of the four conditions will exist at the time you plan to exercise. Increase the odds you'll follow through by attempting to have as many of the four conditions present as you can.

#1 – Pleasure

Human Nature: *We are drawn to what we enjoy.*

It's easy to get ourselves to do the things we enjoy. When we know an activity is going to be fun, it's not a struggle to get ourselves to do it. This is why your exercise program ideally includes the physical activities you most enjoy. Enjoyment of the activity itself is the best of all motivators.

The number of choices for how we could be spending our time at any given moment is unlimited. Since we couldn't function if we considered all of them, we give ourselves a relatively short list of activities to choose from at any given time. We establish different mental lists during different parts of our day. For example, we may have different lists for before work, during the workday, before dinner, after dinner, and just before bedtime.

Although the list we choose from changes throughout the day, the options on our list at a given time are usually fairly consistent from day to day and certain activities tend to compete repeatedly with one another during a particular time slot. For example, the early evening hours may find the recurring competing activities of cooking dinner, watching television, checking social media, and going for a walk. Exercise (in this case, going for a walk) becomes a priority over the other choices when we think we'll enjoy it the most.

> "People rarely succeed unless they have fun in what they are doing."
>
> **Dale Carnegie**

Chuck is a guy I know who isn't really interested in fitness yet still plays on his company's softball team. I was curious to learn more about why he joined the team. He explained that he likes softball and gets to play first base, which is his favorite position. He likes the times during a game when he feels like a hero, having batted in a run or made a good catch. And the competition gets him charged up. Even though he doesn't otherwise get any real exercise, he doesn't feel exhausted after playing. In fact, he says he goes home feeling great. He also likes feeling more connected with the other guys from work.

He shared that his normal after-work routine is to plop down in his recliner and watch the six o'clock evening news. Now, a couple of times a week, he instead goes to a softball practice or game. The choice between going out to play softball and going home to watch television is an easy one. In his case, exercise wins because he enjoys it more.

> "Life must be lived as play."
> **Plato**

Softball is far from an ideal conditioning activity, but that's not what's important. The important thing is to have fun while being active. In addition to providing an enjoyable activity today, softball may well serve as Chuck's gateway to other physical activities. Running a marathon was the farthest thing from my mind when I first started running, but as my enjoyment of running grew, so did my interest in running a marathon.

Life would be wonderful if the pleasure of PREP was all we needed, if the fun we expected from physical activities was always seen as greater than the alternatives. Unfortunately, our favorite activities are often impractical on a daily basis. For example, a kayaking partner of mine, Jennifer, just loves to kayak. She says she enjoys the sensation of gliding across the water and always feels tranquil and peaceful as she paddles along. When she is on the lake, all her worries melt away as the water charges her with positive energy. Jennifer lives too far from the lake to drive there during the week so she jogs after work a couple of days a week to help keep in shape. Since she doesn't enjoy it nearly as much as kayaking, she relies more heavily on the other aspects of PREP—routine, energy, and people—in order to stay consistent with jogging.

If, like Jennifer, you also rely more heavily on the other aspects of PREP, it's still important that you find ways to make your workouts more pleasurable. There are several ways you can do this.

Try exercising in a setting that appeals to you. Although I enjoy jogging in my neighborhood and admiring people's homes and yards, it pales in comparison to how much I enjoy jogging on the path that winds along the river. The river and trees are beautiful. Wildlife, including squirrels, deer, foxes, and geese, is everywhere. There is no auto traffic, just other people out on foot or on their bikes enjoying the great outdoors. The activity is the same, but the setting makes the experience very different.

Adding music is another good way to make a workout more enjoyable. Movement and music just naturally go together—crank up your favorite upbeat song and see if you can sit still. Technology has made it easier than ever to have your favorite music playing while you are on the move.

The good news is that once you're able to gain some consistency, you'll naturally develop more enjoyment of your physical activities. It's not uncommon for an activity that doesn't start out high on our fun-scale to evolve into something we enjoy. Often, it takes time before we connect with its own particular joy. Ask a runner how much she enjoyed running when she first started. Most likely, she'll admit that in the beginning she felt running was a mundane activity worthwhile only because it would help her lose a few pounds. Over time, however, she developed a connection to it and now experiences running as a peaceful communion with nature and self that clears her mind and nourishes her soul.

After I graduated from college and finally successfully implemented a regular fitness program, I started with running. So that I could compete in triathlons, I later took up cycling. In the beginning, I had a clear preference for running over cycling. But over the years, I grew to love cycling; after about a decade, I finally came to the point where I enjoyed them equally.

> "When you're curious, you find lots of interesting things to do."
> **Walt Disney**

The more physical activities you can find that you enjoy, the better. Is there a sport you have been curious about but never tried? Give it a chance. An open mind and an adventurous spirit are priceless.

You may also find that the more fit you become, the more interest you have in other activities. For example, a writer friend, Carol, wasn't exercising and was unfit by any standard. She wanted to lose some weight and decided she was going to start walking. After gradually building up to relatively long walks, she decided to try hiking, too. Now she's in a hiking club and hikes regularly.

Pleasure is a strong motivator. So put the power of pleasure to work for you. Do activities you like. Make them fun.

#2 – Routine

Human Nature: *We are creatures of habit.*

Studies have found that somewhere between 40% and 90% of our behavior is driven by habit. Hard to believe? Think of your morning routine. How much does it vary from day to day? Notice the consistency in what you do, the order in which you do it, and the time spent on each activity. Since it would be incredibly time-consuming to document everything you did during the day based on habit, instead note the amount of time spent doing things you don't normally do. Notice what a small percentage it is of the 24 hours available to you. It will become clear that doing something unique is the exception and not the rule. It's important to recognize that our lives are governed by our daily routines and that we need to harness the tremendous power that habits exert over our lives.

> "A habit is something you can do without thinking — which is why most of us have so many of them."
>
> **Frank A. Clark**

Although our habits limit us, they also serve us. They allow us to function with less thought and energy. The body can be busy showering and getting ready for work while the mind is miles away thinking of the day ahead or that upcoming vacation. Routines allow us to go onto autopilot. If we successfully turn exercise into a habit, we'll do it without even taking the time to decide if we want to or not. We just do it automatically.

> "Men's natures are alike;
> it is their habits that separate them."
> **Confucius**

Unfortunately, it takes time to develop a habit. Research on how long it takes to develop a habit has produced varied results because so many variables have an impact, including the degree of change from current behaviors, motivation level, activity frequency, and techniques employed to help encourage the habit. The most frequently cited length of time is 21 days, but my personal observation is it takes longer than this for exercise to become a habit. This causes the other elements of PREP to be even more important when beginning a new exercise program.

It's easier to establish a new habit if it's linked to an existing habit. For example, mealtimes tend to be strongly habitual (I'm a big fan of eating everyday), and can, therefore, be a good anchor for a fitness habit. Many people exercise just before breakfast, lunch, or dinner. Exercising after meals will work, too, if you do activities such as walking or cycling which are not too jarring. This approach has the added benefit of making the meal more enjoyable, knowing it's feeding a workout rather than your waistline.

Maintaining an exercise program is much easier once it becomes part of your normal routine. Yet, although habits are strong forces, they are not foolproof. Many people who were initially doing great sticking with established exercise programs find themselves no longer exercising after a vacation and don't understand why. The problem is that the habit was broken. The routine has to be reestablished, and like in the beginning, they need to rely on the other elements of PREP until the habit takes root again.

#3 – Energy

Human Nature: *Our energy level fluctuates throughout the day.*

It takes energy to initiate physical activity. This is the law of inertia, Newton's first law of motion that we learned back in grade school. It states that a body in motion will stay in motion, while a body at rest will stay at rest, unless it is compelled to change state by an applied force. This means that to get ourselves started we need a little push.

Unless we have someone willing to drag us out the door, we need a way to push ourselves. Since we cannot physically drag ourselves, we have only one source for that force: energy.

"Energy is the essence of life."
Oprah Winfrey

Those of us living in the Western world typically don't pay too much attention to our energy. We focus more on our thoughts and feelings. We notice how our body looks and functions with very little attention given to the force that drives it.

Our bodies must produce energy in order to survive. Movement stimulates the body's production of energy. To better understand the importance of movement to energy, try this experiment. Lie perfectly still. After 15 minutes, notice your energy level. Afterwards, go for a 15-minute walk and then again assess your energy level. It should be noticeably higher.

Our energy level fluctuates throughout the day, but tends to follow a recurring pattern from day to day. We often consider ourselves either a "morning person" or a "night person," having noticed a pattern of highs and lows. Chart your energy level on an hourly basis for a few days and without fail you'll see a distinct daily pattern emerge.

Knowing your energy pattern is vital because doing something that requires self-discipline requires energy. You may have had the experience while dieting that you stuck with your diet for most of the day, but gave into temptation later on in the evening. For many, this is the time when energy—and, therefore, willpower—is the lowest.

Your willpower won't be strong enough to get you started in a workout if your energy is too low. Therefore, it's important to schedule workouts as often as possible during those times when your energy level will be high. This is especially true before exercise has been transformed into a habit, since the energy demand is higher.

> "Life is energy, if it is anything."
> **Napoleon Hill**

It won't always be possible to time your workout with a high-energy state. Furthermore, your typical energy patterns can easily be thrown off on any given day. A lack of sleep, a heavy meal, or encountering a major disappointment are just a few examples of things that can drain your energy level. The people around you have an impact, too. We all know "energy vampires" who use their toxic mix of gossip and negativity to suck the life force right out of us.

For this reason, it's important to learn those things that will quickly raise your energy level high enough to get yourself moving. For some, it could come from consuming something to raise blood sugar levels a bit, such as drinking some juice. For others, it may come from something that makes them laugh. The right music can get us charged up. Deep breathing exercises can stimulate energy. Sunlight can help.

> "Energy creates energy. It is by spending oneself that one becomes rich."
> **Sarah Bernhardt**

Since movement stimulates energy production, do some mild stretching or walking to get activated. Generating your own energy is similar to generating power with turbines below a dam. It takes some energy to initially open up the intake gates to start the flow of water over the turbine blades that gets them spinning. The turbines don't instantly generate power, but it's not long before the flow of the water has them spinning faster and faster, generating more and more energy. Similarly, it doesn't take long for our bodies, once put into motion, to generate a surplus of energy beyond what we are using. Five or 10 minutes are all it takes. Physical activity is the original renewable energy source.

By way of example, I'm happy to share a couple of my personal routines for combating a low energy state. If at home, I start by drinking some type of fruit juice. Next, I lie on the floor with my legs propped up on a chair. Having my legs elevated allows the blood to drain to my torso and head. This takes the pressure off of my legs and helps them to feel less fatigued. The extra blood supply to the rest of my body helps me to feel more energized. Allowing my muscles to relax also helps. After 10 or 15 minutes, the combined effect of all of these factors is sufficient to raise my energy level enough to get myself out the door and doing the planned workout.

If at work, I am able to raise my energy level sufficiently by simply drinking some hot chocolate. While I'm aware it's not exactly health food, it's worth it if it helps make my workout happen. It also has the benefit of adding some water into my system and warding off hunger if my stomach is empty.

In addition to raising my energy level, these practices also help me leverage the routine aspect of PREP discussed in the previous section. They are part of an established pattern. After I complete them, I get up and go. Having a preprogrammed sequence, whether with a rocket launch or a workout, makes it easier to get moving.

> "Our fatigue is often not caused by work, but by worry, resentment and frustration."
> **Dale Carnegie**

Try to anticipate days and situations that may alter your normal energy pattern. Interpersonal conflicts can significantly drain us. Feeling overwhelmed, stressed, guilty, or envious will deplete energy. We often know in advance when we will experience situations that will cause these types of feelings. Recognize this and adjust knowing you may not have your normal energy level at that time.

Also take note of other recent changes in your life requiring additional self-discipline. Have you started a new diet or committed to some other resolution? If too much is doled out for other purposes, we'll lack the energy needed to overcome inertia to get ourselves to exercise.

#4 – People

Human Nature: *People care about other people.*

Most of us are responsible adults. We have learned the importance of being responsible, so we act that way the majority of the time. We've all had irresponsible actions come back to haunt us.

But let's face it. We also know in the short run life is easier when we are irresponsible. If nobody else is impacted, it's easier to just go with what's easy. Forget being responsible. After all, you're responsible all day long. Who's it going to hurt if you skip today's workout? Right?

Our commitment to exercise actually does affect others. Exercise improves our mood and ability to handle stress.

In short, we are more enjoyable for others to be around. It helps to recognize that our decision to exercise does affect others because we'll sometimes do things for others that we won't do for ourselves. We clean the house when we're having company coming over. We slave over the stove to make others happy with a satisfying, homemade meal. We'll endure great personal sacrifice to see that our family members are safe, healthy, and happy.

Seeing your exercising as a benefit to others can encourage you to do it. Take a moment to consider who else might benefit if you were to exercise regularly.

- Who would you set a good example for?

- What things might you do for others if you had more energy?

- Who would benefit if you felt less stressed and were in a good mood more often?

- Who would be happy knowing you were taking good care of yourself?

Jack and Ken are a couple of recently retired guys from my local business community. In talking to them before their retirement, both spoke with conviction of big plans to start exercising now that they would have so much more time on their hands.

When I ran into Jack a couple of months later he admitted he'd not been doing much exercising. He said that even though he was retired, he was still having trouble finding the time; the weeks had been busier than he had anticipated. He hoped to find time "when things settled down a bit." Odds are not in his favor.

When I met up with Ken about a month after that, he proudly reported he had been sticking with his exercise routine. I, of course, complimented him and asked what things were contributing to his success. One of the things he mentioned was his grandson, Michael.

Ken has been babysitting Michael on Friday afternoons since retiring. Ken explained that when he babysat Michael before retiring, he hadn't really engaged with him. "I spent most of the time just sitting in my chair, watching Michael play with his toys or watch videos."

He also shared that having been very driven and committed to his career as a real estate broker, he'd not spent as much time as he should have with his own kids while they grew up. It wasn't too uncommon for him to miss his kids' games or cancel family outings so he could show a home or close another deal.

He said he was determined to be a better grandfather than he was a father. A big part of his commitment to exercise was that he just loved Michael and wanted to have the energy to be an active grandfather for him. He said, "I don't want Michael to remember me as that gray-haired old man who just sat in his recliner."

> "Example is not the main thing in influencing others.
> It is the only thing."
> **Albert Schweitzer**

To increase your commitment to staying fit, consider the benefit to others. If you have children or grandchildren, consider the impact that not exercising has on them. In a study involving 4,000 schoolchildren, University of Essex researchers found that children who reported that their parents do almost no physical activity were 50% more likely to be unfit than children with more active parents. A study published by the *Journal of Pediatrics* found children with one active parent were 3.5 times more likely to be active themselves and children with two active parents were 5.8 times more likely to be active themselves.

Kids take a lot of energy. Without the additional energy developed by exercise, it's tough to have the energy needed to play and engage with kids in a meaningful way. Many people become so worn down by daily life that there is nothing left for the most precious thing of all, quality time with their children. They muster just enough energy to make them behave and keep them out of their hair. Nobody plans for this to happen, but without exercise it often does. Imagine how much better things would be having as much energy as kids do.

My neighbors Robert and Jan began exercising for the sake of their dog, Mimi. After their veterinarian explained that Mimi's health was suffering from a lack of exercise, they began daily walks with her. Now, they wouldn't dream of Mimi missing her walk. They actually needed the exercise for their own health as much as Mimi's, but never made it a priority. In fact, they still view the walks as Mimi's fitness program even though they've both lost weight and feel noticeably better.

An American Heart Association study found people were 76% more likely to take a walk if another person was counting on them. We don't like to disappoint people. If we are no-shows, we know it will have a negative impact. Our workout partner may skip their workout because we did. At a minimum, he or she will enjoy the workout less without our company.

Take advantage of this aspect of our nature; you'll find there are plenty of ways to involve others. You could start taking walks with a coworker during afternoon breaks, sign up with a personal trainer for regular sessions each week, commit to taking your child to the park once a week to play Frisbee, or do whatever else appeals to you. Commitments to others reinforce the commitment you've made to yourself.

Putting it Together

Your chance of completing a workout rises as the number of PREP conditions increase, so plan your activities and timing to maximize them at the time of your workout.

I met Candice last year as a fellow volunteer at a local festival. We worked the same booth and during the day I taught her about PREP. When I ran into her at this year's festival, she proudly explained how she had created a Monday night workout that combines all four PREP conditions. Mondays are usually her toughest day at work and she feels a little relieved and uplifted when the workday ends (energy). She has made it part of her routine schedule to drive directly over to her friend Mika's house after work (routine). Candice wanted to help Mika get in shape because Mika needs it even more than she does (people). They enjoy a 30- to 45-minute walk together in the regional park near Mika's house, chatting the whole way (pleasure). Even though sometimes holidays interfere, Candice has found this to be the workout she is most consistent with.

PREP will also help when you're "not in the mood" as the workout approaches. When you just don't feel like working out, go through the conditions list and ask yourself question like:

- How can I make this workout more enjoyable?

- How important is it to keep my exercise habit alive?

- What could I do right now to raise my energy level?

- Who will congratulate me for pushing through?

This questioning moves you from focusing on the problem—*I don't feel like exercising*—to focusing on the solution.

PREP works for more than just exercise. It will work for any healthy habit you'd like to create. For many years I was unsuccessful in maintaining a regular habit of flossing my teeth. Just as people know the benefits of exercise, I knew the benefits of flossing but I still wasn't doing it. Every hygienist I ever met gave me a lecture and eventually, deep scale cleanings became necessary. Anyone who has experienced this procedure without pain medication knows this alone should've been sufficient motivation to keep me flossing for the rest of my life. But, it wasn't.

I would at times become motivated to floss for a while, but it was never long before motivation waned and I stopped. Then it would be months or even years before I built up the motivation to try it again.

> "Insanity: doing the same thing over and over again and expecting different results."
>
> **Albert Einstein**

My approach to flossing was similar to how most people approach exercise. I assumed it was all a matter of invoking self-discipline to force myself to do it. Each time I took the same "just do it" approach despite its previous lack of success. I thought I just needed to try harder. It escaped me how I could have good self-control in other areas of my life and continually fail at flossing.

My use of **PREP** allowed me to finally break free of this repetitive cycle of failure. Once I decided to apply it, I quickly realized using the power of pleasure and people were out. I couldn't see how I could actually enjoy flossing, nor did I see my lack of flossing as hurting anyone else. I could, however, see how I could harness the power of routine and energy. I decided to link flossing to a well-established daily habit: shaving. It stood to reason that if I had time to shave, I also had time to floss.

Previously, my flossing was done just before going to bed. It had seemed logical that the best time to floss was after I was done eating for the day. What I failed to recognize was this was my lowest energy state of the day. My self-control was at its weakest point. It's obvious now why this approach continually failed.

Shifting flossing from just before bed to the morning when I shave had the effect of moving it from my lowest energy state to my highest (I am a "morning person"). The linkage to another habit made it easier to establish flossing as part of my daily rituals. I have had no problem maintaining a regular habit of flossing ever since.

The remainder of this book will provide a more comprehensive look at the factors that will lead to your long-term success in making fitness a regular part of your life. You'll see PREP elements intertwined throughout. We'll be exploring other aspects of human nature you can take advantage of, too.

In the next chapter, we begin by examining your attitudes and beliefs because they ultimately determine your success in any endeavor, including exercise. We'll explore below the surface to identify those things that may have impeded your success in the past and look at how to establish a more supportive mindset. This is a critical component to creating exercise as a natural extension of you.

CHAPTER HIGHLIGHTS

PREP to Exercise
- There are four conditions that help enable exercise: pleasure, routine, energy, and people.

#1 – Pleasure
- It is easier to get yourself to do something if you enjoy it.

#2 – Routine
- Most of what you do is based on habit.

#3 – Energy
- It takes energy to invoke willpower and overcome inertia.

#4 – People
- You will sometimes do things for others that you wouldn't do strictly for your own benefit.

Putting it Together
- The more of the four conditions of PREP that exist, the more likely you are to do a workout.

ACTION STEPS

✔ Memorize the four components of PREP.

✔ List the physical activities you enjoy in order of preference and determine how you could do more of your top choices.

✔ Identify an established habit you could link with exercise.

✔ Identify your daily energy patterns and determine how you could best schedule exercise when in higher energy states.

✔ Experiment to find things that quickly raise your energy level.

✔ Make a list of who beside yourself would benefit from you exercising.

Chapter 3

Your Attitudes and Beliefs

"Nothing can stop the man with the right mental attitude from achieving his goal; nothing on earth can help the man with the wrong mental attitude."

Thomas Jefferson

Capture the BEAR

Human Nature: *We create results that support our beliefs.*

Our lives are governed by our beliefs. Our beliefs determine how we evaluate everything. All we see, hear, smell, feel, or think passes through the filter of our beliefs. It's through our beliefs that we judge the world and our place within it.

"It all depends on how we look at things, and not how they are in themselves."

Carl Jung

Your beliefs determine if you view something as either good or bad. It's easy to find examples of times people responded differently to the same situation based on their beliefs. You may go to the movies with friends and find some loved the film while others thought it was awful. The event was identical. You all saw the same movie at the same time in the same place, but because everyone's beliefs are different about what is interesting, funny, or entertaining, each comes away with different judgments of it.

Your belief system, then, must support what you say you want because you will create outcomes that align with your beliefs. An excellent example is the familiar "placebo effect." People have had astonishing health improvements by taking a pill that contained no medication. They improved because they were told and believed they were taking a drug that had the power to cure them. They were cured solely by their belief. In fact, the impact of the belief system is so well established that scientific studies are now careful to use techniques to help eliminate this factor from the results.

> "Whether you believe you can do a thing or not,
> you are right."
> **Henry Ford**

To successfully create an exercise habit you must first believe it's possible. You must *know* that if you just had the right advice and approach, you could join the ranks of people who exercise consistently. The chart on page 41 illustrates how our beliefs influence our results. Using the acronym, remember, "It's a BEAR to get what you want."

Here's what BEAR stands for:

Belief

Emotion

Action

Result

Beliefs create emotions. Emotions create actions. Actions create *results*.

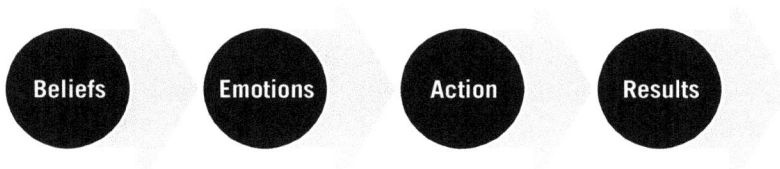

Our beliefs determine how we feel about things, in other words: what we like and don't like. We naturally move toward what we like and away from what we don't like, and this drives our actions. These actions create the outcomes we experience.

> "The greatest discovery of my generation is that a human being can alter his life by altering his attitudes."
> **William James**

Since beliefs are the starting point, it's important to begin by understanding what your beliefs are about exercise. If you believe exercise is an unpleasant chore that's to be endured rather than enjoyed, you will be unsuccessful in making it a habit. Determination will only take you so far.

The good news is that you are free to believe whatever you want. No one can force you to believe something. What you believe is entirely your choice.

> "People will generally accept facts as truth only if the facts agree with what they already believe."
>
> **Andy Rooney**

The problem is we typically forget we have this choice. Most of our beliefs have developed so gradually over time that we rarely question them. Every day we notice the things that support our beliefs and disregard the things that don't. These selective reinforcements build upon each other creating a mountain of proof in our minds that our beliefs accurately reflect reality. Our beliefs have driven our actions producing self-fulfilling prophecies.

Interestingly, it's easy for us to recognize the inaccurate or limiting beliefs of others. For example, you probably know someone with talent that she fails to put to use. She doesn't see her gift as anything special, and as a result, hasn't pursued something that could be life changing. We all have limiting beliefs, but it's difficult to see them in ourselves. It's like trying to see the back of your own head; it takes a lot of reflection.

> "Man is made by his belief. As he believes, so he is."
>
> **Johann Wolfgang von Goethe**

Your Personal Beliefs

Our belief system is the most unique thing about us. We may have the same beliefs about particular topics as others, but no two people have identical beliefs about everything. It's your mental fingerprint, unique only to you. To challenge your beliefs is to challenge your very identity, and that can feel like a violation of sacred ground. The thought of such a challenge can be very unsettling.

But question them you must. Altering beliefs is the only way you'll evolve. Chances are you know people who are "set in their ways" and won't consider changing their beliefs. They're stuck where they are and will never progress as human beings. It's our willingness to challenge our beliefs which provides the opportunity to improve ourselves.

> "When you're finished changing, you're finished."
> **Benjamin Franklin**

Are you set in your ways concerning exercise? Undoubtedly you have beliefs that have obstructed the incorporation of exercise as a natural and enjoyable part of your life. It's critical to determine what those are. Use the questions below to start exploring your beliefs about exercise.

- What pictures or feelings come to mind when you hear the word "exercise"?

- What thoughts and feelings do you have just before heading off to exercise?

- What are your top three positive associations with exercise?

- What are your top three negative associations?

- How do you react when someone talks about his or her exercise regime?

- What thoughts come to mind when you see someone jogging or cycling along the road?

- When deciding if you will do a workout, what images come to mind and how do you expect it to feel?

- What are you predominantly thinking about and feeling during a workout?

Your answers will help identify what you associate with exercise. Use these clues to gain insight into your beliefs. Write down your beliefs to help you stay conscious of them. Use what you learn as you progress through this book to help reinforce the positive ones and to challenge and change those that are negative.

It's also helpful to understand where your beliefs came from. Think about your exercise history going clear back to childhood:

- Did you look forward to P.E. in school?

- Did you compete in a sport?

- Were the experiences generally positive or negative?

- How did your relationship with exercise develop over time?

> "I have memories—but only a fool stores his past in the future."
> **David Gerrold**

We've all had some type of negative experience with exercise. You may have tried to get in shape doing an activity you didn't enjoy or you overdid it and ended up incredibly sore, injured, or burned out. You need to stop negative associations, including those developed long ago, from defeating your attempts to enjoy exercise. Determine which ones are interfering. The first step in eliminating the power of the past is recognizing its grip. The past no longer exists anywhere but in your mind. It can only impact your future if you allow it to do so.

My friend Rita had been struggling for quite some time to become consistent in going to her health club. When I posed these questions to her, she had the following response: "When I think of exercise I picture myself struggling in the class I do. Beforehand, I'm slightly dreading it, knowing it's going to be hard."

From discussing her answers, we were able to uncover her belief that she was failing if she didn't keep up with everybody else in the class. She believed that exercise was not doing her any good unless she pushed herself to the point of feeling quite miserable.

We easily find excuses in order to avoid something unpleasant. We don't like to be miserable and we don't like to feel like a failure. Rita realized this is why she had been finding excuses to avoid going to the gym.

She hadn't fully understood how much the proper activity level varies from person to person or even how much it varies for any given individual. A 20-mile run may be a good workout for a marathoner training for a race and a completely ridiculous workout for that same runner when recovering from a race or injury. After identifying the beliefs that were holding her back, Rita came to see that what other people can do or being able to push through a set class length weren't good measures of success or failure.

Rita bought a heart rate monitor and found she isn't miserable when she maintains her intensity within an appropriate range. Now she gives herself permission to do less than others if necessary to keep her activity at the right level for her.

Because she took the time to uncover her faulty beliefs and address them, she now looks forward to and enjoys her classes. When Rita changed her beliefs, she changed her results.

Self-Image

Human Nature: *We act in accordance with how we see ourselves..*

We have countless beliefs about people, places, experiences, concepts, and a host of other things. The beliefs that exert the most significant control over our lives, however, are the ones we have about ourselves. Collectively these beliefs are known as our self-image.

Our self-image guides what we will and will not do. If I see myself as having a good sense of humor, I'll crack jokes. If I see myself as someone who is uncomfortable in front of a group, I will avoid leading discussions, making presentations, or engaging in any other activity that makes me the center of attention. If I see myself as someone who doesn't enjoy exercise, I'll find ways to avoid it.

Your self-image affects the type and amount of exercise you'll do or if you'll even exercise at all. Part of how my friend Lisa stays in shape is by going to a Zumba® class at a dance studio. She enjoys the class, but hasn't been going as consistently as she would like. In using my advice to increase the number of PREP elements she has working for her, she attempted to get a buddy from work, Joann, to start going with her. She and Joann are good friends and she knew Joann would like the class, too. Yet no matter how much Lisa tried, she couldn't get Joann to try it.

> "It is what a man thinks of himself that really determines his fate."
>
> **Henry David Thoreau**

Joann used to be very petite when she was younger and having added some pounds over the years, now has a distorted view of herself as a monstrosity. She eventually explained to Lisa that when she thought of going to the class, she got cartoon images in her head of a dancing hippo in a pink tutu. Lisa assured her that there were other women in the class larger than her, but it didn't matter. Joann just couldn't seem to see it any other way. It's a shame because, had she gone, she probably would have enjoyed the class and done well having a friend to go with. But her self-image held her back.

Nothing is more fundamental to success in living an active lifestyle than a honed self-image as an active person. Exercise must be the natural result of the kind of person we are, rather than merely an activity we choose to do sometimes and not to do at other times. How do you see yourself when it comes to fitness?

- Are you unsure why you have had trouble sticking with exercise, or do you know it's because you are just not the type of person that can?

- Do you ever call yourself a couch potato?

- Do you see yourself as someone who doesn't enjoy exercise?

- Do you think you have the wrong personality to become a regular exerciser?

- What do you assume other people are thinking about you as you exercise?

- How do you describe yourself to others when it comes to fitness?

> "We will act consistent with our view of who we truly are, whether that view is accurate or not."
> **Tony Robbins**

These are important questions because what we consistently think and say about ourselves ultimately becomes true. If you see yourself as someone who does not enjoy exercise, on a subconscious level your brain will work to see that this belief holds true. You'll focus on everything about it that could be seen as unpleasant. You'll look for reasons why you can't exercise rather than ways you could. Conversely, if you see yourself as someone who enjoys exercise, opportunities to feel alive and engaged with the world through physical activity will constantly spring up.

It's difficult for us to do something which conflicts with our self-image. It's like riding a bicycle whose handlebars won't turn. We can lean hard and make slight changes in direction, but we will be unable to make significant changes in the direction we're headed. The further away your self-image is from that of an active person, the more difficult it will be to steer yourself onto that path.

> "It does not manifest so that you can believe in it. You believe in it so that it can manifest."
>
> **Lauren Zimmerman**

You're not doomed, however. As with other types of beliefs, what we choose to believe about ourselves is our choice. A person who sees himself as lazy can decide to see himself as an active individual. Since acting inconsistently with our self-image is always short-lived, if he sincerely and consistently holds this new belief, it will, in fact, become true.

Sound simple? In theory, it is quite simple. In reality, though, not so much. The problem lies in the process of changing beliefs. Our conscious mind wants proof of a new belief before adopting it. Unfortunately, we have difficulty obtaining this proof because our subconscious mind works to reinforce whatever our current beliefs are. It's a Catch-22. The new belief won't be true until you believe it and you won't believe it until it's true.

> "We must walk consciously only part way toward our goal and then leap in the dark to our success."
> **Henry David Thoreau**

Changing beliefs, then, requires a leap of faith. Make that leap. Recognize that limiting beliefs are paper tigers. Decide now that you are someone who is dedicated to fitness. There is no reason not to believe it. The past is in the past. You don't have to define yourself by past failures to stay in shape. Study anyone who has achieved greatness and you'll find he or she had many failures—usually big ones—before triumphing. You can achieve great things, too, if you, like them, define yourself by your successes rather than your failures. At this moment you're taking the time to read and learn how to achieve your fitness goals, so you'll be successful in achieving them. Accept this as proof you're a person committed to fitness.

Use Pictures

To support your view of yourself as an active person, start picturing yourself this way. The more often you do, the more quickly it will become true. While still in bed, spend a few moments picturing yourself enjoying the physical activities you'll do during the day. Find other moments during your daily routine to picture yourself being active. See yourself doing specific activities and getting specific pleasure out of them for specific reasons. The more frequently and vividly you picture yourself being active, the more likely it is to happen.

> "Hold a picture of yourself long and steady enough in your mind's eye and you will be drawn toward it."
> **Napoleon Hill**

An especially powerful time to create mental images of yourself being active is as you're relaxing to fall asleep. This is because it's highly effective in planting the image in both the conscious and the subconscious parts of the mind. Both control our behavior, so the impact is multiplied. Studies have found that the majority of regular exercisers, while waiting to fall asleep, picture themselves exercising.

It encourages your identity as an active person if your surroundings reinforce it. Do you have pictures you could put on your wall, desk, cell phone wallpaper, or computer screensaver of a time you felt good while being physically active? Find pictures of a ski trip, playing in the yard, a team photo, or any others that remind you of a happy time while being active. These visual cues will help reinforce your identity as an active person. The pictures around us help create similar pictures in our minds. The pictures held consistently in our minds are ultimately created in reality. Picturing yourself as a person who enjoys being active is critical in making it so.

Body Image

Our self-image includes how we view our bodies. We tend to judge our bodies based on how they compare to what we view as ideal. We are far more likely to compare ourselves to a model than a sumo wrestler, so the comparisons we choose usually make us unhappy with our bodies. We spend far more time focusing on what we don't like about our bodies than on what we do like.

We treat well that which we love and cherish. If we don't love our bodies, we're less likely to do what's good for it. I have many times heard people say they hate their body. Consider how you treat the things you hate compared to the things you love and you'll understand the importance of loving your body unconditionally.

Does your body have flaws? Of course it does. I have yet to meet the person who wouldn't change something if he or she could. Do you only love people without flaws? Of course not. We all love imperfect people, so why would we not also love our imperfect body? The human body is the most amazing creation on the entire planet. We are extremely lucky to have one! So what if yours doesn't look like others? How boring would it be if everybody were identical? The human body is not a curse. It's the greatest gift we could possibly have been given.

Belonging

An indicator of our self-image is the type of groups we feel we fit into. Do you see yourself as belonging with the fitness enthusiasts group? Since the majority of the population doesn't exercise consistently, the people who do are, by definition, abnormal. Many people take shelter in the idea that by not exercising they're normal. There is a temptation, even, to think there is something wrong with the people who do exercise. It's easy to stereotype the exercisers as "overachievers" or "masochists" and, therefore, not a group we fit in with.

"Life isn't about finding yourself. It is about creating yourself."
George Bernard Shaw

Realize that the group that is "into" fitness is far broader than those diehards that religiously work out at least an hour every day. The truth is the fitness crowd includes people with a wide range of activity levels. Regular exercisers come from all walks of life and include every personality type imaginable. The woman who works up a sweat pushing her baby in a stroller around their neighborhood is just as much a part of the fitness movement as the marathoner. There is no set amount of exercise you must do to be a fitness enthusiast. It doesn't matter how much exercising you've done in the past or what kind of shape you're in now. As long as you have a desire to be active and fit, you're part of the exercise community. There are no membership applications, dues, or initiations. Membership to this group is instant; you belong the moment you believe you do.

"Instead of worrying about what people say of you, why not spend time trying to accomplish something they will admire."
Dale Carnegie

Often overweight or out-of-shape people feel awkward walking into a gym surrounded by fit-looking individuals. They feel out of place and assume others are thinking they don't belong. If you ever find yourself in this position, recognize these are your thoughts and not those of the people around you. In almost any situation, what people are thinking is rarely as bad as we assume. People who exercise are always happy to see another person join the ranks. Additionally, people are much more likely thinking about themselves and what they are doing. The others in the gym are more concerned with their own workout than they are with whether or not you belong. If they do happen to pay attention to you, they are most likely admiring your commitment to make a change.

Self-Worth

Human Nature: *We treat well that which we value.*

A direct product of our self-image is our self-worth. Our self-worth affects how well we treat ourselves and how we prioritize meeting our own needs against meeting the needs of others.

"No body is worth more than your body."
Melody Carstairs

Finding time to exercise is usually part of this balancing act. It's important we be aware of how often our opportunity to exercise is lost in order to meet someone else's needs. We are in charge of our health and happiness; no one else can provide this for us. If we constantly sacrifice ourselves, we need to explore why the importance of our own health and happiness is so low.

There are times when skipping a planned workout for someone else's benefit is absolutely the right thing to do. If this happens routinely, however, it calls your level of self-worth into question. If the demands consistently come from the same person, it calls into question the value he or she places on your health and happiness. Consistently choosing not to work out in order to please someone else benefits no one in the long run.

"Whoever is happy will make others happy too."
Helen Keller

Some people see exercise as a selfish act. They have trouble balancing it against the demands of their job or family. The fact is both your employer and your family benefit enormously from your exercising. You are more alert, productive, energetic, patient, and optimistic when you are fit. It helps you to be a better worker, parent, and lover. Taking the time to exercise is not selfish. What is selfish is someone who interferes with the healthy habits of others for his or her own benefit.

Definition of Old

Human Nature: *We are only as old as we think we are.*

Do you limit yourself by seeing yourself as old? You probably have a predetermined number that defines old, such as turning 30, 40, or 50. You drastically lower your standards and expectations for your physical abilities when you think of yourself as old.

The symptoms of aging and inactivity are nearly identical. People often chalk up the decline they see in their physical abilities strictly to aging. Research has found that the decline in the body's capabilities due to aging is a fraction of what people generally believe. The fact is most of the physical decline we experience in the passing years is a reflection of how well we have been taking care of ourselves rather than the natural aging process.

> "We don't stop playing because we grow old; we grow old because we stop playing."
> **George Bernard Shaw**

We speed up the aging process by not getting enough exercise. A research team from Stanford University followed more than 4,300 initially healthy people over the course of 20 years. The level of fitness the subjects maintained turned out to be the best predictor of mortality. The mortality rate for the people that were least fit was twice as high as the second-least-fit group of people and four times as high as the most fit. Many other studies have also shown a positive correlation between fitness and longevity.

Equally important are the findings that fitness not only adds years to life, but quality, too. In a study of the records of 18,670 participants spanning 40 years, researchers from UT Southwestern Medical Center and The Cooper Institute found the onset of chronic diseases occurred much later for those individuals who were fit during midlife.

Not surprisingly, then, a study conducted by the K.G. Jebsen Center of Exercise in Medicine of 4,631 healthy individuals from age 20 to 90 found age is much less important than activity level in determining fitness. Their findings suggest than an active 50-year- old can be just as fit as a less active 20-year-old.

> "To be 70 years young is sometimes far more cheerful and hopeful than to be 40 years old."
> **Oliver Wendell Holmes**

Jack LaLanne has been called "The Godfather of Fitness." He opened the first health club in America and had a nationally televised fitness program for 30 years. He once said, "People don't die of old age, they die of inactivity." At age 70, he pulled 70 people in 70 boats for 1.5 miles in Long Beach Harbor while handcuffed and shackled.

Jack LaLanne is far from being the only example of how capable a body kept fit remains. In 2005, Robert McKeague of Villa Park, Illinois, successfully completed the Hawaii Ironman Triathlon in 16 hours 21 minutes and 55 seconds. This race entails a 2.4-mile ocean swim, 112-mile bike ride, and 26.2-mile (marathon) run. It's done in the heat, humidity, and wind of Hawaii and is considered to be the toughest single day sporting event in the world. Robert was 80 years old at the time of the race.

And at age 98, Keiko Fukuda became the first woman in history to earn a tenth-degree judo black belt.

> "Everyone desires to live long, but no one would be old."
>
> **Abraham Lincoln**

There are countless other examples of people who have chosen to stay fit, and, as a result, stayed physically vibrant. Increasingly, people are beginning to realize that becoming older doesn't mean growing old if fitness is maintained. Fortunately, you don't have to have been a fitness fanatic all of your life to get the health benefits. It's less important how old you are when you start; what matters most is that you stick with it once you begin.

I knew a woman who at 102 years of age would say, "I'm getting old." Most of us would say she had already gotten there! Yet I believe her viewpoint was part of why she lived so long. She didn't see herself as old; she was only on her way.

It's true that you are older now than you've ever been. It's equally true that you're younger now than you'll ever be! Rather than choosing to feel old, decide to take advantage of your relative youth. Adopt a definition that old is at least 20 years older than you are right now. Allow your definition of old to roll up a year each year. This way you won't even be old at age 90. It will be those people who are 110 who are old!

Personal Responsibility

Human Nature: *We are more committed to solving problems we own.*

It's easy to blame circumstances for causing us to fail. After all, life is full of surprises. It's also full of people who place demands on us and try to influence how we spend our time. It's tempting to attribute a missed workout on a situation or other people. For example, I could say I didn't exercise today because my boss made me work late. I feel better knowing that it's not my fault.

> "We can let circumstances rule us, or we can take charge and rule our lives from within."
>
> **Earl Nightingale**

But I am really just fooling myself. I know the nature of my job and should've been able to predict my boss would ask me to work late today—or at least at some point. It's not my boss's responsibility to never ask me to work late. It's my responsibility to anticipate and be prepared for it with a backup plan ready for when it happens. I should know in advance how I'll adjust my normal routines or revise the type of exercise I'll do in order to still do a workout.

Life is a continuous stream of choices. You can't control every outcome, but what you did or didn't do always contributes to the result. You'll get what you want only when you take the time to identify your role in getting the results you didn't want.

A relative of mine has been overweight his entire adult life. He says, "I was born this way; I was a fat baby." He scoffs at exercise and maintains an unhealthy diet, yet doesn't see himself as having a choice in being overweight. Ironically, he is disgusted by people who are more overweight than he is. It's easier to recognize dodging personal responsibility in others than in ourselves.

Think of someone you know who doesn't take responsibility for his or her actions. Is this person happy? Is he or she successful in meeting meaningful goals? Do you wish you were more like this person? Probably not. Taking personal responsibility is a fundamental ingredient to achieving results that make your life happy and fulfilling.

> "The majority of men meet with failure because of their lack of persistence in creating new plans to take the place of those which fail."
>
> **Napoleon Hill**

Carefully scrutinize situations when circumstances caused you to miss a workout. Could you have seen those circumstances coming? Have they happened before? Are they likely to happen again? What can you do to prevent them from happening again? If they do happen again, how can you adjust so your workout isn't missed? The number of options you find will be directly proportional to your level of commitment.

Even worse than allowing circumstances to disrupt your fitness goals is allowing them to be a complete barrier to ever beginning. You may be tempted to wait until an upcoming event, obstacle, or obligation is behind you before you begin exercising. "I'll wait until after the holidays when things aren't so busy" is a common excuse.

Yet life is a never-ending series of events, obstacles, and obligations. You may like to believe that your life will lack demands and challenges at some point, but the unfortunate reality is, it never will. The nature of your challenges will change, but they always exist in one form or another. That's life. If exercise only occurs when circumstances are perfect, exercise will never occur. The only successful strategy is to solve the challenges that arise and develop skill in exercising in spite of them.

Expectations

Human Nature: *We have good days and bad days.*

Your beliefs, associations, and self-image are deeply ingrained. You have the power to change them but need to understand that the process will take focused effort and energy. You can make immediate progress, but continued reinforcement is necessary to make changes permanent.

When you attempt to make changes in yourself and your life, be prepared for self-doubt because it always accompanies significant change. Accept it as a normal and natural part of the change process that happens to everyone.

"Doubt is not a pleasant condition, but certainty is absurd."
Voltaire

When self-doubt shows up, greet it as you would a needy friend who has yet again shown up on your doorstep at the worst possible time. When those thoughts of doubt enter, be gracious, but not overly welcoming. "Hello, Doubt, I have been expecting you. I am sorry, but our visit will have to be short. I have other commitments."

This may sound a little silly, but what's really silly is to allow self-doubt to stop you from getting what you want. Doubt only has the power you give it. You can't avoid having negative or defeatist thoughts pop into your head, such as "Who am I kidding? I'll never be able to stick with this." You're bound to experience this at least occasionally, but you're not obligated to accept it. You have a choice. Would you allow the needy friend to stay indefinitely and make your life decisions for you? You couldn't prevent the knock on your door, but how the visit affects your life is entirely your decision.

Recognize that this time really *is* different. You're taking the time to learn how to be successful. You're unearthing your past mistakes and acquiring the knowledge necessary to develop a better approach. Usher your doubts out to the street to find someone else to bother.

With your new knowledge and approach, it will be far easier to establish and maintain a habit of exercising. This isn't to say it will be easy forever more and you'll never think twice about doing your planned workout. Getting yourself to exercise is a learned skill. As with any new skill, you improve as time goes on. As your new approach to exercise becomes more familiar, it becomes easier. Don't allow doubt back in the door because of early struggles you have with developing your perfect formula.

Daily Fluctuations

Not all days are created equal. Expect that as with anything you do frequently, there will be good days and bad days. You experience a constantly changing mixture of conditions in life. Your stress level, emotional state, and energy level in addition to the amount of sleep you've had, emotional state of the people you interact with, and weather are just a few of the variables that are in constant flux. This can impact how easily you get yourself to do a workout or how you experience it.

> "Our greatest glory is not in never falling,
> but in rising every time we fall."
> **Confucius**

Accept this as normal, natural, and unavoidable. Don't allow an off day to be an excuse to quit. We don't quit our job because of a tough day, send our children off to boarding school when they become challenging or quit watching movies because we sat through a crummy one. Even professional athletes have off days. We've all seen it: the unstoppable athlete who crumbles during an important game or competition. They keep going because they're paid to, and while you may not draw a paycheck for your efforts, remember that you have a payoff, too. When you continue to make exercise a part of your life, the payoff is infinitely more valuable than money. Your health and vitality improve.

Patience

Too often people hold exercise to a higher standard than the other essentials in life, expecting it to always be a breeze or fun. But let's face it. Having a job or caring for a family isn't always easy or nonstop fun, yet we still do these things and generally find them valuable parts of our lives. With the right approach, exercise will frequently be the best part of your day. On those days when it's not, take pride in your perseverance.

Many enter into an exercise routine with unrealistic expectations of how quickly they will see results. The demand for instant gratification rules today's society, and as a consequence, many find the gradual nature of improvements from exercise disheartening.

Exercise shouldn't be adopted as a quick-fix solution. And anyway, how often is the quick answer the best? Some of the benefits of exercise are immediate, while others can take a great deal of time to become apparent. Take comfort in the knowledge that the longer you continue to exercise, the more you'll benefit from it. Results are inevitable.

To build a house that will stand for many years to come, we must start with a solid foundation. Similarly, building fitness as an enduring structure in our lives begins by creating a solid foundation of the supportive attitudes and beliefs presented in this chapter. In the next chapter, we'll address motivation, which, like the nails and joists of a house, holds our fitness structure together. People who quit exercising often cite lack of motivation as the reason. We'll explore how to stay motivated and avoid falling prey to losing interest in exercise.

CHAPTER HIGHLIGHTS

Capture the BEAR
- Your beliefs influence your results.

Self-Image
- Seeing yourself as a fitness enthusiast leads to being more active.

Self-Worth
- Exercise becomes a higher priority the more you value yourself.

Definition of Old
- How "old" you feel is greatly determined by how active you are.

Personal Responsibility
- Your actions, not your circumstances, create your outcomes.

Expectations
- Self-doubt and off days are a normal part of the change process.

ACTION STEPS

✔ List negative associations related to past exercise experiences and how they came about.

✔ Write out positive beliefs you'll adopt to replace the negative ones you've been hanging on to. Post them in a visible place where you will be reminded constantly of them.

✔ Alter any views that might keep you from now seeing yourself as a fitness enthusiast.

✔ As you are falling asleep at night, or when you first wake in the morning, create mental pictures of being active.

✔ Change your computer screensaver and cell phone wallpaper to pictures of yourself being active and happy.

✔ Become aware of when self-doubt enters your mind and practice kicking the negative thought to the curb, immediately replacing it with a positive one.

Chapter 4

Get Motivated!

———◄———

"Continuous effort—not strength or intelligence—
is the key to unlocking our potential."

Winston Churchill

Valuation of Benefits

Human Nature: *We will do that which
makes us feel good.*

Everything we do is done to benefit us in some way. Exercise is no exception. It's done strictly for the positive results it produces. If exercise were bad for us, we would all avoid it.

Motivation for any action is directly tied to the value we place on the expected outcome. The more we desire the results, the higher our motivation. Offer me $5 to mow your lawn and you won't get much response. Offer me $1,000 and I'll be right on it!

For this reason, identifying the benefits you hope to realize from exercise is the starting point in maximizing your motivation level. I'm sure you're aware of what you hope to gain. If you're like most people, you want to lose weight. Some will start for health reasons, though usually only after something significant has happened, such as the diagnosis of a medical condition that exercise could help address.

It's important to also identify less visible results you would like to see by exercising. The idea of being thinner or having better vital signs is not usually a strong enough reason to sustain motivation over the long haul. To maintain the long-term motivation needed to exercise regularly, you need to understand how you'll *feel* better having these results.

> "The starting point of all achievement is desire."
> **Napoleon Hill**

Bring to mind the picture of yourself in the future after you have become fit. What do you imagine it will be like? Will you feel more attractive and desirable? Will you feel less self-conscious when meeting new people? Do you see a more powerful and confident person? How good will it feel to stand in front of a mirror and smile because of what you see? How much more will you enjoy a piece of chocolate cake knowing you'll simply burn it off? How much joy will you feel fitting into clothes that had become too small? Will you feel healthy and relaxed? Do you see a more energetic person?

"If you plan on being anything less than you are capable of being, you will probably be unhappy all the days of your life."

Abraham Maslow

It's not the idea of losing 20 pounds that will get you out of bed an hour earlier to fit in a morning workout. It's being able to be the person you want to be and feel the way you want to feel. Create vivid pictures of this more vital version of you and what it feels like. Imagine how much happier you'll be. Allow the passion for becoming this person to flow through your veins. Remember that emotions drive your actions and fuel your motivation. An intellectual recognition that exercise will have some good outcomes isn't enough. You must have strong feelings about it. The bigger the change you want to make in your life, the more you'll need to be emotionally invested in the desired outcome.

Valuing the full spectrum of benefits exercise has to offer will help further fortify your motivation. Review the list of benefits below and rate the value of each.

Scale: 1 = Not Important 5 = Utmost Importance

		1	2	3	4	5
1.	Promotion of weight loss	1	2	3	4	5
2.	Maintenance of a healthy weight	1	2	3	4	5
3.	Lowered risk of heart disease	1	2	3	4	5
4.	Lowered risk of cancer	1	2	3	4	5
5.	Lowered risk of stroke	1	2	3	4	5

6. Lowered risk or severity of diabetes   1   2   3   4   5

7. Lowered blood pressure   1   2   3   4   5

8. Lowered cholesterol level   1   2   3   4   5

9. Improved immune system function   1   2   3   4   5

10. Stronger bones   1   2   3   4   5

11. Stronger muscles   1   2   3   4   5

12. Larger muscles   1   2   3   4   5

13. Increased flexibility   1   2   3   4   5

14. Stress release & increased relaxation   1   2   3   4   5

15. Better night's sleep   1   2   3   4   5

16. Improved energy, stamina & vitality   1   2   3   4   5

17. Endorphin release & improved mood   1   2   3   4   5

18. Improved ability to concentrate & focus   1   2   3   4   5

19. Improved problem solving & creativity   1   2   3   4   5

20. Increased opportunity to enjoy nature   1   2   3   4   5

21. Enjoyment of competition   1   2   3   4   5

22. Increased opportunities to socialize   1   2   3   4   5

23. Improved body image   1   2   3   4   5

24. Improved self-esteem & confidence   1   2   3   4   5

25. Increased sense of accomplishment   1   2   3   4   5

Consider getting a physical examination if it has been awhile since your last one. Discuss your blood pressure, resting heart rate, blood sugar, blood lipids, and body fat levels with your doctor. You may discover you have a condition or health risk that you weren't aware of which exercise could help alleviate. Your motivation to exercise will rise significantly the moment that it becomes real how exercise will specifically impact how long and well you'll live.

Identify Costs

Human Nature: *We recoil in the face of unexpected costs.*

As is often said, nothing in life comes for free. The best time to recognize the cost of anything is before it needs to be paid. Many have failed to stick with their exercise program because the costs weren't adequately anticipated.

> "For everything you have missed, you have gained something else, and for everything you gain, you lose something else."
> **Ralph Waldo Emerson**

The monetary costs are usually the easiest to identify, but these are rarely the most important. Exercise doesn't require that you spend money. It does require, though, that you spend time and energy; this is where most fail to make the necessary investment.

Consider the cost of exercise:

- Who will you end up spending less time with?

- What will you have to stop doing?

- What will you have to start doing?

- What will be given up?

Use these questions to help determine your cost to exercise. List the costs (undesirable results) you anticipate in the chart below and rank the importance.

Scale: 1 = Not Important   5 = Utmost Importance

1. _____ 1   2   3   4   5

2. _____ 1   2   3   4   5

3. _____ 1   2   3   4   5

4. _____ 1   2   3   4   5

5. _____ 1   2   3   4   5

6. _____ 1   2   3   4   5

7. _____ 1   2   3   4   5

8. _____ 1   2   3   4   5

Cost/Benefit Analysis

Human Nature: *The bigger the payoff, the more we are motivated.*

A cost/benefit analysis is far from a new evaluation technique. It has been used in business for about as long as humans have been conducting business. It's still in use today for good reason; this technique makes it clear if something makes sense to do or not. It simply entails comparing the costs of doing something to the benefits. If the costs outweigh the benefits, you don't do it. If the benefits exceed the costs, you do.

Review the benefits and costs of exercise you identified in the previous two sections. Is exercise worth it? On balance, how much will exercise create an improvement in your life? If you see your life becoming worse or only slightly better, you'll lack sufficient motivation to exercise. It's only when you recognize exercise will create an overall significant improvement in your life that you'll invest the time and energy it takes.

The good news is that the longer you stick with exercise, the more of the benefits of exercise you'll experience. Beyond the physical changes, you'll start to recognize mental and emotional improvements. For example, you'll notice you're better able to concentrate and you have more patience. Also, over time, you'll learn ways to work it into your life with less sacrifice. All of this helps to tip the scales even further toward a continuing commitment to exercise.

Accountability

Human Nature: *We prefer the feeling of success over failure.*

If we feel responsible for something, we feel good when we are successful in achieving it and feel bad when we're not. This is why many attempt to shift responsibility in the face of failure. Feelings of failure can be avoided by blaming other people or "unforeseeable circumstances." If I can convince myself a failure is not my fault, I don't have to feel bad about it.

"He that is good for making excuses is seldom good for anything else."
Benjamin Franklin

We don't like to feel bad, so playing the blame game is quite a temptation; however, it doesn't serve us well. We are solely responsible for our fitness. No one else is capable of the job. Any success or failure is ours and ours alone. Success will not be achieved without accepting full responsibility. Owning this accountability allows the full force of the positive and negative feelings of success and failure to drive your emotions and, therefore, your behavior.

For accountability to exist there must be a measurable outcome. Accountability is created by assigning responsibility in a manner that allows objective measurement as to whether or not a responsibility has been met. In other words, it allows success and failure to be objectively determined.

> "There are two primary choices in life: to accept conditions as they exist, or accept the responsibility for changing them."
> **Dennis Waitley**

For example, I may be responsible for helping keep the house clean. If this responsibility remains general and undefined, a clean house and the adequacy of my contribution are subjective judgments that leave success and failure open to debate. I could do very little while still claiming to have met my responsibility. If, on the other hand, I am made accountable for sweeping the floors every other day, taking the trash out twice a week, and dusting the furniture weekly, my success or failure can be measured. I need to do all of these activities to claim success in meeting my responsibility.

A familiar axiom in business is "What gets measured gets done." Of course, it's not the act of measuring that produces the results. It's the accountability that the measurement fosters. Measure the amount of exercise you do to create accountability and increase motivation. The amount planned and achieved need to be routinely compared.

Competition

Human Nature: *Our competitive spirit drives us to excel.*

Our society is schizophrenic when it comes to its views of competition. Top competitors in sports and business are celebrated and awarded huge salaries, yet it's not uncommon for people to be chastised for being competitive. Many people are embarrassed to admit they are competitive because it's so often judged as a negative trait. Paradoxically, competition underlies the laws of nature, and therefore, nothing could be more natural.

Being able to compete successfully is fundamental to success in virtually all aspects of our lives. We must beat the competition to get a job, a promotion, or win customers. We need to compete for the affections of that certain someone and with all of life's distractions to maintain a close family.

> "You can discover more about a person in an hour of play than in a year of conversation."
> **Plato**

A competitive spirit can be a priceless asset in becoming fit and staying that way. It's not something to be ashamed of. The desire to excel is something to be cultivated, not squashed. It just needs to be properly channeled. Embrace any competitive nature you have and put it to work for you.

My friend Nicole was having trouble getting back into an exercise routine. Since some of her friends were having the same problem, they decided to band together for a 30-day fitness challenge. They created a competition to see who could log the most miles walking, running, and cycling over the course of the 30 days. Each committed $25 that would be donated to the charity chosen by the winner.

Nicole was inspired by the friendly competition and wanted her charity to win so she started logging miles right away. She began looking for reasons and places to ride her bike. She went for hikes on weekends. She logged some type of miles almost daily for the month. Her friends were also ignited by the competition and were far more active than they had been.

The competition was good for the entire group (not to mention the charity!). Consider if you could create some type of friendly competition with people you know. You'll be doing everyone a favor.

"Games lubricate the body and the mind."
Benjamin Franklin

The world of fitness is loaded with opportunity to engage in healthy competition. Virtually every sport has competitive events. These can be very strong motivators for competitive types. Even people who are not especially competitive find enjoyment in the special sort of camaraderie that comes from being part of a team.

A downside to being competitive is that it can be difficult for highly competitive types to get into a new sport. It takes time to become skilled and initial performances will reflect this. The desire to perform well compared to others can override the urge to try something new or reenter a sport when substantial fitness has been lost.

One cure is recognizing that competition doesn't have to be against others. There are plenty of ways for us to compete against ourselves. Motivation can be found in breaking our own records for distance, speed, or gracefulness.

"None are so old as those who have outlived enthusiasm."
Henry David Thoreau

By nature, even those who consider themselves non-competitive are inspired by challenges. You may have heard the familiar saying, "Why does a man climb a mountain? Because it's there." Conquest is part of our instinct which drives us to climb to that mountaintop. The challenge we normally seek to conquer may only be to see if we can go a little longer or a little faster, but it's the same force that propels us. Think of a time you set a challenge for yourself and then were successful in achieving it. It felt good, right? Exercise is loaded with opportunities to feel uplifted in triumph. Tap into this primal drive and then enjoy the glow of victory.

Guide Your Focus

Human Nature: *Our focus determines our experience.*

At any given moment there are countless things we could potentially notice. We tend to think we thoroughly observe most of what's going on in our body and environment, but in actuality we can't possibly pay attention to more than a fraction of it. Look around the room. It's filled with objects you weren't paying attention to. Is there a picture that's not perfectly level? Is there dust you didn't immediately see? Can you smell anything? How comfortable is your sitting position? Do you have any body tension or aching muscles? How do your toes feel? How deeply are you breathing? The things you could be paying attention to at this one moment in this one room are astronomical.

> "What we see depends mainly on what we look for."
> **John Lubbock**

Imagine if every time you wanted to eat at your home you gave no thought to how good the food would taste and how much you would enjoy the meal, but instead only focused on the burns you might receive handling hot pots and pans, the ache in your legs that might arise from standing on the hard kitchen floor, and the certain drudgery of scrubbing the dishes afterward. What if in deciding to dine out, instead of thinking about the delicious choices on the menu, you focused on the gas-guzzling slog through traffic to the restaurant, the potential germs that might be passed along from those preparing and serving the food, and the fact that you would be opening your wallet while knowing it was unnecessary that you spent your hard-earned money this way? How much would you enjoy your meals?

To most, this may seem like an unusually pessimistic way to think, yet this is precisely the mindset many people take with exercise. Instead of thinking about the many benefits they'll receive from exercise, they just focus on the aspects they don't like. And focusing on the wrong things can make otherwise good experiences miserable. A former coworker once told me he wouldn't want to win the lottery because he would then have to pay a lot of taxes. Don't share his attitude and spoil exercise by focusing on the wrong aspects.

> "Men are not prisoners of fate, but only prisoners of their own minds."
> **Franklin D. Roosevelt**

There are plenty of positive aspects to focus on, such as improved health, increased vitality, but most importantly, the joy you can find in an individual workout. As important as the long-term benefits are, exercising only for the sake of an eventual outcome, like weight loss, is a missed opportunity to maximize our motivation.

Long-term exercisers have one thing in common. They appreciate the long-term benefits of exercise, but this isn't usually all that drives them to do a day's workout. In addition to the long-term benefits, they know they'll also get something out of it that very day. They find enjoyment or recognize a good outcome nearly every time they work out.

By doing so, they're working with their human nature; we naturally prefer instant gratification. Doing something today that will benefit us sometime in the future is simply not as compelling as doing something that will benefit us today. This will never change. Exercise has a high dropout rate because people often start exercising for the future benefit of looking better or improving their health, yet these benefits appear gradually. We all have limits in the amount we are willing to sacrifice today for future gain, and many people reach their limit with exercise before the benefits they're looking for make much of a showing.

> "In the end, it's not the years in your life that count. It's the life in your years."
>
> **Abraham Lincoln**

On the other hand, getting instant results and enjoyment never gets old. From the outset then, you need to recognize the immediate benefits. If you find it hard to imagine experiencing any immediate benefits while exercising, remember that how we experience anything can be changed by altering our focus. We pay attention to stimulus based on our habits unless our attention is somehow directed otherwise. If, like many, you have the habit of focusing on the things you don't like about exercise, try to make a habit of noticing the positives in your exercise experience. These positive aspects can be found from three categories: the environment, the activity, and the immediate results.

Environment

Enjoy your surroundings when you exercise. If you look for beauty, you will surely find it. You may find it in nature, such as flowers, trees, rivers, lakes, or a beautiful sky. You may encounter appealing man-made structures like fountains, bridges, or attractive homes. You may see uplifting activities as you pass by—a family playing tag together in the park, for example, or a young child giddy with the joy of riding a bicycle. Notice nice fragrances from the trees and bushes or simply take pleasure in breathing fresh air into your lungs.

Enjoy the sound of birds singing or the rustling of the wind through the trees.

> "Everybody needs beauty as well as bread, places to play in and pray in, where nature may heal and give strength to body and soul."
>
> **John Muir**

Finding beauty in the world nourishes the soul. Connecting with nature feeds an important part of us that has shriveled in our technology-driven world. Many psychologists encourage a regular connection to nature as an aid in maintaining good mental health. Enjoying the outdoors while working out can help keep you whole and healthy.

While in my opinion nothing compares with nature, you can make indoor environments enjoyable, as well. Put on music you like or listen to an audiobook. Position yourself to have a nice view out of the window or where you can watch a program or video you'll enjoy. Add some personality to your workout space. Be creative.

Activity

Find enjoyment in the activity itself by savoring the emotional highs and the pleasant sensations created by movement. For example: The rhythmic motion and breathing from swimming or the concentrated exertion from lifting weights can feel amazing. There's satisfaction in learning to master an activity that requires concentration and skill, such as martial arts. You may enjoy the thrill of rock climbing or kayaking. You may get a charge from the competition of playing basketball, volleyball, or tennis or you may simply have fun interacting with others.

> "We think too much and feel too little."
> **Charlie Chaplin**

There are many ways to enjoy your activities. Identify what appeals to you and make it part of your focus while you exercise.

Immediate Results

Enjoy the immediate results delivered by exercise. It can make you feel better in a variety of ways. It's a great way to release tension and help you feel more relaxed. It can create an endorphin release within your body which will improve your mood. It activates your body's energy production which will leave you feeling recharged and invigorated. It can also provide a sense of pride, accomplishment, and self-confidence.

> "Rejoice in the things that are present;
> all else is beyond thee."
> **Montaigne**

After you exercise, notice how much better you feel. Make sure to take a moment to revel in the good feelings that came from exercising.

Focusing on elements from each of these three categories will greatly improve your enjoyment of exercise. And once you find the joy in exercise, it will completely change how you relate to it. Just as eating healthily is not a chore when the food tastes good, exercise is not a chore when it feels good. Your long-term success is dependent upon finding exercise enjoyable on a daily basis. Recognize and appreciate all of the good things exercise provides each and every time and you'll come back to it again and again.

Read

The more you think about something, the more it becomes part of you and your life. So spend time reading about your chosen activity. Books are worthwhile because they can provide in-depth information and uplifting success stories, but magazines (or ezines) can at times be even better because they provide a constant stream of easily digestible new material. Publications cover general fitness as well as every imaginable activity. The price of a subscription is a tremendous value considering the amount of information they provide, including how to lower the risk of injury, technical information on how to perform better, product reviews, new approaches to keep things interesting, similar activities you may enjoy, upcoming events, success stories, and general tips and support.

> "What we think, we become."
> **Buddha**

A magazine can help serve as a coach, providing you with the information and inspiration needed to keep going. Activities will be more enjoyable as you become more knowledgeable, skilled, and confident. Regularly reading about the activity will help maintain your focus and deepen your connection to it.

Also make a habit of reading articles or blogs that talk about the benefits of exercise as a way to constantly feed your commitment. These are plentiful on the Internet allowing you to easily create a steady diet of exercise information and motivation.

Slogans

Marketers know they must get people to remember and identify with their brand and products so they often utilize a jingle or catchphrase. It's easy to recall a long list of advertising slogans we're familiar with because they stick with us. Their catchiness is why corporations spend billions of dollars on them and you've been hearing them all of your life.

Harness the power of slogans for yourself to increase your focus on exercise. Create your own, link it to a positive image, and repeat it as much as possible to increase its effectiveness. For example, my friend Tim regularly says to himself, "Fit is fun." When he says it, he pictures himself enjoying soccer with his friends. A paired slogan and image like this have to be believed to have an impact. In Tim's case, he's convinced that he wouldn't enjoy soccer if he weren't fit. His slogan maintains his focus and reinforces the value placed on exercise.

> "You affect your subconscious mind by verbal repetition."
> **W. Clement Stone**

My personal slogan is "swim, bike, run" repeated three times through in fast succession. I know it may not sound too engaging, but it works for me. It came about from my early years of exercise when I focused primarily on competing in triathlons. Come up with a good one for yourself. Your slogan can develop substantial power over time in keeping you connected to fitness.

Like most thoughts, my slogan just pops into my head seemingly out of the blue. When I had a running injury and decided to take up kayaking to replace running, I gave my slogan a twist: "swim, bike, *row*." Despite this being only a slight change, I couldn't make it. Swim-bike-run would automatically pop into my head so fast, my conscious mind didn't have time to stop and edit it. After months of trying, I resigned to leaving it unchanged. That's the power of a slogan.

Our experiences in life are guided by what we pay attention to and focus on. We become that which we consistently think of becoming. Keep your focus on those things that support your interest and desire to exercise. Make this focus a habit and your exercise habit will surely follow.

In these past two chapters, we have explored how to prepare your mind and adjust your thinking in order to make regular exercise part of your life. This is where it all starts, but it doesn't end there. There is more you can do. You increase your chances of success by also cultivating your social environment.

This is done by engaging the people around you and identifying others who can contribute to your efforts. You may already be aware of how people around you have affected your intention to exercise in the past. We'll explore this dynamic in greater depth. The next chapter will guide you through this, in addition to outlining how to create a system of social support which will contribute greatly to your achieving the results you want.

CHAPTER HIGHLIGHTS

Valuation of Benefits
- The benefits of exercise have the most motivational power when you understand how they will make you feel.

Identify Cost
- Everything, including exercise, comes with some sort of cost.

Cost/Benefit Analysis
- Comparing the benefits of exercise to the costs makes its value clear.

Accountability
- Measuring exercise activity is necessary to create accountability.

Competition
- Competitive drive can be harnessed to help you become and stay fit.

Guide Your Focus
- Your focus determines your exercise experience.

ACTION STEPS

✔ Identify the most important ways exercising will make you feel better.

✔ Determine how you can reduce the negative impact of taking the time to exercise.

✔ Consider ways you might leverage your competitive spirit to help create a more active lifestyle.

✔ Determine the enjoyable aspects you'll focus on for the exercise you'll do.

✔ Select a magazine to subscribe to or a blog to follow.

✔ Create your personal exercise slogan.

Chapter 5

Gain Social Support

"You can't make positive choices for the rest of your life without an environment that makes those choices easy, natural, and enjoyable."

Deepak Chopra

Enlist Your Social Circle

Human Nature: *We are affected by those around us.*

For better or worse, the people around you influence your intentions to be fit. Some people are direct and obvious, such as a spouse who strongly protests against investing in a gym membership. Some are subtler—for example, a close friend who says, "People should learn to age gracefully and not do all that silly hopping around."

It has been put this way: you are the average of the five people you spend most of your time with. While this overstates the case a bit, it does point to the value of taking a look at those around you and noticing how they influence your desire to be fit. Nobody operates in isolation; each of us interacts with others, whose words and actions either encourage or discourage us. The amount of passion they have for either our success or our failure will affect us. The impact upon us depends on how much we value their opinions and on our relationship with them.

> "Be careful the friends you choose
> for you will become like them."
>
> **W. Clement Stone**

Even if you're surrounded by negativity, you may not realize it. What seems normal and natural to you is based on how you were raised and the people you have surrounded yourself with since then. Use the chart below to objectively evaluate the composition of your present social circle.

Write people's names that fit each description & category below:

Description	Family	Friends	Boss & Coworkers	Neighbors & Acquaintances
Makes negative comments about exercise or the people who do it				
Has complained about an inconvenience created by my exercising				
Criticizes or discourages me when I exercise				

Description	Family	Friends	Boss & Coworkers	Neighbors & Acquaintances
Seems to feel threatened by the idea of my becoming fit				
Gives me reasons or temptations to skip workouts				
Exercises as part of his or her lifestyle				
Regularly talks about physical activities he or she enjoys				
Encourages or praises me when I exercise				
Does or may be interested in doing physical activities with me				
Willingly makes adjustments that make it easier for me to exercise				
Knows when I am or am not meeting my fitness goals				
Encourages me or provides rewards for sticking to my exercise plan				
Has helped me make improvements in other areas of my life				
Has a more positive attitude towards life compared to most				

From completing this chart it should be apparent who the positive and negative influences are. Determine who around you will be supportive and who is likely to impede your fitness efforts.

Develop Your Team

Fitness is a team effort. To create your own personal team, you'll need a coach, cheerleaders, and supporters.

Coach

Not that long ago, hiring personal trainers was only for the rich and famous. Over time, though, more and more people have come to recognize the value of having a coach, and hiring personal trainers is now common among "ordinary people." The instruction, structure, and inspiration trainers provide can make a big difference in staying fit.

There are various coaching options. You can hire a personal trainer who works at your health club, find one who makes house calls, or find an online trainer who does his or her coaching remotely using the Internet. There are also virtual coaching options available using software applications.

It's not absolutely necessary to hire a coach, but it helps to at least have some type of mentor. Mentors greatly increase our chances for success in any new endeavor, and maintaining a regular exercise program is no exception. If you know someone that has been successful in staying fit, see if this person would be willing to take you under his or her wing. A good coach or mentor can be a tremendous help in coming up with ideas for overcoming the barriers that inevitably arise and in getting to the root of potential struggles you may face, like missing workouts.

If you're not immediately able to hire a coach or find a mentor, at least recruit a friend or family member who is willing to hold you accountable and call you out when you're making excuses rather than finding solutions.

Cheerleaders

It's amazing how much easier a difficult task can become when you have someone cheering you on. This is constantly demonstrated in sports, but it applies to most areas of our lives. I'll bet you can think back to a time someone encouraged you and it made a big difference.

Cheerleaders can be anyone providing encouragement and applauding your efforts and successes. This requires very little commitment from the person, so hopefully you can surround yourself with lots of them.

Supporters

Undoubtedly, you have many obligations and demands on your time. Even the most organized and dedicated among us find it difficult to fit in exercise without a little help sometimes.

Supporters are the people that help us with logistics that make fitness more easily fit into our daily lives. For example, a supporter could be a boss who allows you to work flexible hours or a spouse willing to watch the kids or cook dinner when you would otherwise.

From your evaluation of your social circle, identify who might fit into each role and enlist their support. People are far more likely to provide you with the support you need if you tell them exactly what you need or want from them. They must also know what your exercise plans are. The more concrete the plan, the more prepared they will be to support it. Here are the points you will want to cover in your discussion:

- Why you're committed to regular exercise

- What your exercise plan entails

- Their role and importance in your success

- Their willingness to support your efforts

- How much you'll appreciate their support

Fitness Partners

Human Nature: *We like to share experiences with others.*

We have all heard the saying that misery loves company. Well, so does fun! Think of the fun things you do and how many of them you prefer to do with others. Do you generally prefer to go to the movies, go out to dinner, see a performance, or take a trip with others or alone? We have a natural tendency to enjoy experiences more when someone is enjoying it with us. This also applies to exercise.

The degree to which we enjoy socializing varies from person to person, but we all have a need for social contact and support. Exercise can be a rewarding and rejuvenating solitary experience, but even the most reclusive types can find enjoyment in occasionally sharing the experience. We are social creatures by nature. The lone runner is not really alone, because she is often thinking of conversations and interactions with other people while her legs churn away. She is kept company by all those people in her head traveling along with her.

> "Success comes when people act together;
> failure tends to happen alone."
> **Deepak Chopra**

Finding the right person or group of people with whom to share your exercise experiences is of tremendous value, and even more so if you can recruit a family member. Studies conducted by Indiana University found that married couples that worked out separately were six times more likely to quit within a year than those couples who exercised together. Additionally, sharing interests and activities strengthens relationships. There is a good reason for the saying, "A family that plays together, stays together." Sharing in a physical activity provides a strong bonding experience. If there is someone you would like to build a deeper relationship with, consider finding a way to engage in some sort of exercise together.

There is a synergistic result from working out with a partner. The energy we generate while we exercise feeds each other, creating more enthusiasm and resolve for both. Partners can help one another overcome the challenges faced with staying fit; this is especially valuable if you haven't enlisted the support of a coach or mentor. Sometimes it takes out-of-the-box thinking to solve problems, and since we *are* the box, we need the help of others to provide fresh ideas to conquer our challenges. Our partners can also make all the difference in getting us going when we are struggling with an off day, and it's a good feeling when we are able to return the favor.

Pets can make excellent fitness partners. Dogs, for example, can provide added safety as well as companionship, along with the satisfaction of knowing we are doing something good for them, too. And it's easier to get ourselves out the door when we see how excited our dog is to go out.

Personal trainers can also be fitness partners because they share the exercise experience with us. We have a commitment to them to show up, and we know they'll be disappointed if we don't. It's also a motivator for many people that they'll have to pay for the session regardless of whether they show up. For these reasons, people will often show up to a training session when they wouldn't have otherwise because of their commitment to their trainer.

Find as many fitness partners as you can. To increase your network of partners, consider joining a club centered on running, cycling, hiking, or whatever activity interests you. Most clubs welcome new members and beginners. You'll find the motivation and enthusiasm of other club members is contagious—it's no accident I was in peak condition when I was president of a triathlon club. At the time, my work demands were extreme, but my involvement in the club made all the difference.

Another great place to find fitness partners, even if only for the day, is at a fitness class. Studies have shown a positive influence from having people around us exercising, even if we are not directly interacting with them. Find a class that is well matched with your current fitness level to gain the most sense of connection. It helps to be surrounded by people in a similar phase of fitness to be reminded you're not alone. This sense of community and belonging is powerful in creating a positive attachment to exercise. Attending classes will also provide you with several other benefits, such as:

- A designated time committed to exercising

- Guidance from a trained instructor

- Variety, as routines within a class often vary

- The simplicity of simply showing up and following along

- A dedicated space designed for exercise

- A mental break from focusing on life's problems

- Encouragement from others

Naturally, the more supporters you have in your quest to be fit and the greater their influence upon you, the better. Building and fortifying your support network will be an important factor in your success. Fortunately, the Internet and social media makes it easy to find and connect with others interested in fitness.

As a kid you enjoyed playing with your friends. Keep yourself young by doing the same as an adult. Share the fitness journey and see how much more fun you have.

Heroes

Human Nature: *We are inspired by our heroes.*

Throughout our lives, we come across people we admire because of the type of person they are, what they have accomplished, or what they are able to do. Sometimes it's someone we know or have met, and other times it's someone we don't know personally, such as someone famous or someone we have read about. In any case, they can have a positive impact when we find ourselves inspired to try to be more like them.

Are there people you admire for their physical accomplishments? If so, claim them for your fitness heroes. If no one comes to mind to be your hero, you might consider your personal trainer, if you have one. They almost always have developed excellent attitudes and healthy habits worthy of aspiration. You can also try reading about a sport that interests you. In your reading, you are likely to find some inspirational people. Some may inspire not for the competitions they have won, but for the extraordinary challenges they have overcome.

Shad Ireland is a good example. At age 10, Shad was diagnosed with kidney failure. He then suffered through a decade of dialysis and two failed transplants. Doctors had told him he would probably live to about age 25. Can you imagine being told this at a young age? Essentially, he was just waiting to die.

He saw a televised broadcast of an Ironman Triathlon race (2.4 miles of swimming, 112 miles of cycling, and 26.2 miles of running) and found himself inspired. He decided he was going to do one. In addition to kidney failure, he had cardiovascular disease and blood pressure issues. At 75 pounds and unable to walk on a treadmill for 30 seconds, the likelihood of completing the triathlon was not a long shot; the idea was completely absurd.

Through sheer guts and years of perseverance, he eventually went on to become the first dialysis patient to complete an Ironman Triathlon. Shad has continued to participate in marathons, triathlons, and cycling events despite having had to hook himself up to a dialysis machine for over 30 years. Besides serving as an incredible living example of hope and possibility, he raises money through his foundation to help others affected by kidney disease.

One of my heroes, and the hero of many others I know, is my friend Byron Sliger. At five feet eight inches tall and 293 pounds, he used to be anything but the picture of health. Besides never exercising, he lived on junk food, smoked two packs of cigarettes a day, and regularly drank enough beer to intoxicate a moose. Then, it happened. He was diagnosed with cancer.

With great determination he decided he was going to defeat cancer by changing his life to become fit and healthy. He quit smoking, excessive drinking, and changed his diet. He began running. He lost over 100 pounds and completed a marathon. It was my pleasure to coach him for his first triathlon. He showed up to every training session with a positive attitude and never allowed his treatments or condition to be a reason to back away from the day's workout challenge.

With his new healthy habits, 16 rounds of radiation, and five rounds of chemo, he beat back the cancer. Through it all, he continued to train and race. After several years of remission, the cancer came back. His answer? Endure more treatments and do an ultramarathon race. Again, he successfully defeated cancer and he continues to be an inspiration for many.

While their stories are often not as dramatic as these two examples, all long-term exercisers have had to overcome obstacles and challenges. In the face of these, the stories of inspirational athletes like Shad and Byron can help provide a new perspective. Our own mountain of a problem can shrink down to a molehill when we learn what others have been able to do under far more difficult circumstances.

> "Tell everyone what you want to do and someone will want to help you do it."
>
> **W. Clement Stone**

Modeling, or copying other people who can do what we wish we could do, is a fundamental component of learning. Do you know someone who exercises consistently whom you could emulate? People who have achieved a fitness lifestyle are usually happy to share their enthusiasm and advice, so don't hesitate to ask for pointers. The truth is you'll be helping them while they help you. Allowing them to share their experience and knowledge reinforces their own commitment.

Make a habit of regularly asking others who exercise how their last workout went. They'll be happy to tell you and appreciate your interest. You'll develop a closer relationship with this person and you'll each feel increasingly drawn to exercise.

Events

Human Nature: *We are social creatures.*

Many people have successfully increased their level of commitment by deciding to participate in an organized event. Most communities have annual walking, running, cycling, and triathlon events—you may be surprised to find how many are available once you start looking. Also consider events outside of your immediate area, which let you combine travel with your fitness passion. Is there a well-known event you would feel proud to say you participated in?

> "Goals allow you to control the direction of change in your favor."
> **Brian Tracy**

Having a tangible event to work toward can be very powerful in maintaining motivation. Deadlines help create results. The event serves as a deadline by which time you need to be in sufficient shape to complete it. You will achieve greater consistency with that reinforcement. Consider whether in school you'd have ever studied if there were never tests. The event serves as a test of sorts and will encourage you to do your homework, i.e., the necessary conditioning. Paying the event fee and any associated travel costs in advance can also add to your motivation and commitment.

In addition, athletic events make great opportunities to find good role models or fitness partners. Other people inspire us. Even highly self-motivated individuals draw inspiration from others. Put yourself in an environment where that can happen. A woman I know went to a triathlon merely as a spectator. A stranger walking by said to her, "You look like someone that could do one of these." That passing comment sparked a flame. Despite not really knowing how to swim, she signed up for a triathlon the next day and completed it eight weeks later.

Allowing yourself to be inspired by people in the moment of their exhilaration will also help you see yourself as part of the fitness community and remind you that you are not alone in your fitness journey. Events also encourage you to share concrete goals with your fitness partners. You can agree with a fitness partner that you are both going to participate in a particular upcoming event together. This will reinforce, for both of you, a commitment to prepare.

Events have another significant motivational aspect. They are wonderful social events with positive atmospheres and an almost instant sense of fellowship. You aren't going to find yourself surrounded by a bunch of jocks. Sure, you'll find some very fit people in attendance, but for the most part, you'll discover a diverse group of people spanning a wide range of sizes, shapes, ages, and fitness levels. Rarely will there be a shortage of people you can relate to and connect with, which makes it easy to make new friends.

If you'd like to make an event even more social, try tackling a triathlon as part of a team. Most triathlons allow this option, where different members of the team are responsible for different portions. Do you like to run, bike, or swim? Who do you know that does one of the other two? Being part of a team is both fun and motivational.

There are also events that offer a variety of sports in which you can compete. For example, Corporate Games holds multisport festivals open to every size and kind of organization. Teams can be made up of employees, colleagues, family, and friends, so the events are really open to everyone. Many communities have Senior Games for those aged 50 and over. They are typically multi-day events that offer a variety of sports to compete in, such as volleyball, basketball, swimming, water polo, golf, soccer, softball, table tennis, tennis, racquetball, track and field, cycling, power walking, and running.

Without fail, each athletic event becomes a memorable experience. Completing one usually leads to doing another. In addition to being transformative in their own right, they can provide a real boost in maintaining consistency and enthusiasm in your fitness lifestyle.

Community Service

Human Nature: *We enjoy helping others.*

Some people are more motivated to do a physical activity that produces a result beyond their own bodily health. Performing a "job" is more rewarding to them than something done strictly for the sake of movement. For example, they would be more interested in building a fence than jogging around the neighborhood. They're more inclined to jump on a bicycle if they need to go somewhere rather than taking one to just go for a ride.

Community service can provide endless opportunities to stay fit with activities that accomplish something important. Nonprofit organizations are always looking for volunteers, especially those willing to help with physical labor. Some cities have an organization that matches people looking to volunteer with nonprofit organizations based on their interests. Even without this service, opportunities to volunteer are not hard to find.

> "It is one of the beautiful compensations in this life that no one can sincerely try to help another without helping himself."
>
> **Ralph Waldo Emerson**

My friend Laura volunteers to help build and rehabilitate homes with Habitat for Humanity. This worldwide organization builds homes for people in need through labor from volunteers and the eventual homeowner. Laura has a desk job and these projects help her be more active and fit. The knowledge that she makes a significant contribution to the life of families is a strong motivator, which helps her to welcome the occasional sore muscles. She's always ready to tackle a new project to help another family. Laura recognizes how through this work she has gained commitment, satisfaction, pride, reinforcement, and connection to others. Ultimately, by giving we receive.

Government entities sometimes need help, too. Parks and recreation departments and sheriff offices often have functions manned by volunteers. For example, I help maintain hiking trails in my area by participating in workdays organized by a local nonprofit organization dedicated to this task. I find this to be a great way to combine enjoying the outdoors, getting exercise, meeting nice people, and contributing to my community.

> "Good actions give strength to ourselves
> and inspire good actions in others."
> **Plato**

In volunteering, we gain the satisfaction of knowing we are helping others and contributing to a valuable cause. We can enjoy praise and thanks from the benefiting organization or people we're helping. We meet caring and inspiring individuals from within the community, which deepens our connection to it. There is a special bond created working side by side with those who share a passion to make the world a better place. It allows us an opportunity to recognize the goodness within each other.

Many have become inspired to get in shape so they could participate in a charity walkathon or fun run to help raise funds for a good cause. There are a variety of nonprofit organizations dedicated to research for and treatment of various diseases that have fitness-related programs people can join to help raise funds.

> "What is my life if I am no longer useful to others?"
> **Johann Wolfgang von Goethe**

For example, the Leukemia and Lymphoma Society (LLS) offers a program called Team in Training. In this exceptional program, LLS provides professional training and support for people to complete an endurance event, such as running a marathon, cycling a century ride, or completing a triathlon. The volunteers use their commitment to this major feat as a way to raise funds for cancer research, by asking others to donate based on their physical commitment and the importance of the LLS mission. While raising more than $1.4 billion for cancer research with this program, LLS has also provided training for over 600,000 people who, in the process of helping to save lives, have improved their own fitness and health. In addition, participants have acquired knowledge, skills, and new friends that will help them remain fit—and it all started with their desire to help others.

So far, we've looked at how you can leverage human nature to get motivated and create the best conditions possible for building and maintaining an active lifestyle. Now it's time to get into the details of what that activity might look like. In the next chapter, we'll cover exercise basics. You'll learn how much exercise the body needs, the different types of exercise, recommended intensity levels, and tips on choosing the best activities for you. Knowing the fundamentals is important in all sports, but, as exercise has such an impact on your health, it's even more important to learn the fundamentals for exercise in general.

CHAPTER HIGHLIGHTS

Enlist Your Social Circle
- Fitness is a team effort.

Fitness Partners
- Enjoyment and commitment can be increased by sharing the exercise experience with others.

Heroes
- People we admire for significant or special achievements in sports or fitness can be inspiration for our own stories of triumph.

Events
- Participating in fitness events increases commitment and motivation.

Community Service
- Serving a good cause can add meaning to exercise.

ACTION STEPS

✔ Create your fitness team: coach, cheerleaders, and supporters.

✔ Find fitness partners.

✔ Find fitness heroes.

✔ Select an organized event to participate in.

✔ Find a nonprofit organization you would feel good about providing with free labor.

PART II

Making It Happen

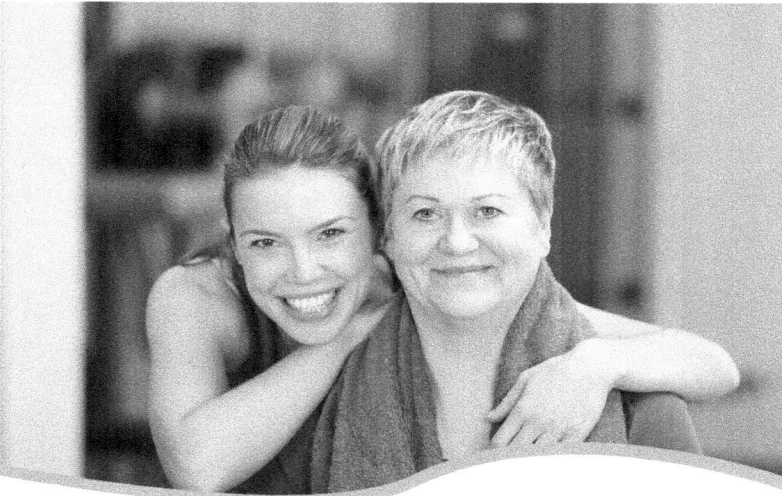

Part II addresses practical matters concerning exercise. We'll discuss in greater depth implementing the concepts presented in Part I and go over fitness basics such as how much exercise your body needs and how to properly plan it. You'll also discover how to further reinforce your motivation, overcome challenges, and deal with slumps. These tools and techniques will make it easier for you to maintain an exercise habit and remain committed to living an active, fit lifestyle.

Chapter 6

Exercise Basics

"Lack of physical activity destroys the good condition of every human being, while movement and methodical physical exercise save it and preserve it."

Plato

Types of Exercise

There are three types of exercise: cardiovascular training, strength training, and flexibility training. The different types of exercise provide different benefits; understanding the primary result of each helps ensure the activities you select can provide the result you are looking for.

Cardiovascular training is often called aerobic exercise. It requires working the body's larger muscles in order to substantially elevate a person's heart rate and oxygen consumption. Examples of aerobic activities are brisk walking, jogging, cycling, and dancing. This type of activity is great for burning calories, strengthening the heart, lowering blood pressure, improving circulation, and lowering cholesterol levels.

Strength training is usually associated with lifting weights. It requires using some form of resistance designed to work the body's muscles. Examples of strength training are lifting weights, pulling stretch cords, and doing isometric exercises like pushups and sit-ups. This type of activity will increase muscle size, which increases the calories we burn even while at rest and allows us to sculpt our form. It also helps with bone density, tendon and ligament strength, and joint function.

Flexibility training is often called stretching. It requires that the body be moved in such a way as to lengthen its muscles. Examples of flexibility training are yoga and tai chi. This type of activity helps keep our muscles supple, which helps to avoid injury. Increased flexibility also helps our normal daily activities, as it makes it easier for us to bend, twist, and reach.

Activity Selection

Matching the primary outcomes you're looking for to the type of exercise you'll do is only part of the equation. There are many paths to get the results you want. Based on the pleasure aspect of PREP discussed in Chapter 2, you want to identify activities you'll most enjoy. The best exercise is the one you'll actually do.

Carley is a great case in point. I often run into Carley at the pool, and recently during one of our brief chats she shared that she has only been a regular swimmer for the last couple of years. She had been on her high school swim team, but didn't continue with any kind of real fitness routine for many years after. Carley came to hate her flabby arms and wanted to make them trim and toned again. When she saw in a magazine a set of exercises she could do using light weights to help tone them up, she started the regime but didn't stick with it for long. A year or so later, Carley began to see advertisements for a rowing machine and just knew it would do the trick. She admitted that using the rowing machine also turned out to be short-lived because "30 minutes on the rowing machine felt like hours."

A few months later, after growing increasing unhappy with her ever-depleting energy, Carley joined a health club with a pool so she could start swimming again. It surprised her how quickly she reconnected with swimming and "started feeling a little more like an athlete and a little less like a soccer mom." She eventually noticed that her arms were starting to "lose their jiggle." This gave her even more desire to keep going to the pool. Now, Carley has more energy and is much happier with how her arms look. She finally got the results she wanted by finding something she enjoys.

Try Something New

Be open-minded and consider activities you may not be as familiar with. There are countless "fringe sports" we don't hear much about, like speed golf or ultimate Frisbee, that may suit you well and make you look forward to your next opportunity to play. Maybe dancing the tango or gyrating with a hula hoop will turn out to be your thing. The potential activities you can do are limited only by your imagination. Look for activities that may be more fun than what you've done in the past and failed to stick with.

"Life is either a great adventure or nothing."
Helen Keller

The more activities you are prepared to do, the easier it is to maintain consistency. For example, team sports can be lots of fun, but typically lack sufficient frequency. Adding in more activities could help with this problem—you could join more than one team, supplement with some other activity you enjoy, or engage in an activity that helps you perform better in your favorite sport. If you like to play soccer, for instance, you could add jogging as an additional activity which would improve your fitness for soccer.

Health clubs have more types of classes to offer than ever with new ones being created all of the time. Be bold. Experiment. Live large. Instructors are eager to help. With an open mind and adventurous spirit, you just might find something fun you didn't expect.

Social Engagement

Consider the activity setting in terms of your sociability. Sports differ in how much involvement with other people they encourage. Racquetball is usually played by two people, golf as a foursome, volleyball with a team of six, and softball with a team of 10. For some, exercise is a great time for quiet reflection, while for others it is a time to enjoy the company of others. For most, a mixture of the two provides the healthiest balance.

Consider who you'd like to spend time with doing an activity. Are there physical activities you might enjoy doing with your child or grandchild? How about a weekly game of badminton or making up a dance routine together? Imagine how good this would be not only for both of you physically but also as a great bonding experience. What could you give them that's more valuable than being able to play with you?

Also consider how much you enjoy competition. Just as sports differ in the amount of socialization they encourage, they differ in their competitive nature. Think about whether you would prefer taking on another team, competing head-to-head, or challenging yourself and your personal records.

Convenience

When striving for consistency, convenience is an important factor to consider. The less logistical hurdles we face, the better. Luckily, there are plenty of workouts that can be done at or near your home. Some of the most convenient options may be exercise DVDs and game console fitness programs, both of which are abundantly available. Most cities have parks which make for great places to get some exercise. Fitness classes and programs can also be found at YMCAs, community centers, community colleges, and churches. Locations close to home, work, or your commute routes are best. Notice if there are any exercise studios you often drive past. Minimize the travel time required to get to the location where you plan to exercise.

Having walking or jogging as part of your activities especially helps maintain consistency because they are so practical. They also provide us the opportunity to enjoy the outdoors and the changing seasons. They don't require other people, extensive equipment, or a special location. A good pair of shoes is all you need. The social aspect can be easily altered from it being a solitary activity to sharing the experience with thousands of others or to anything in between. Plus, walking and running are relatively easy activities to do year-round. During winter, we can add clothing layers or use a treadmill, if we have one available. Your shopping mall may also allow people to come inside to walk before the mall opens.

> "Walking is the best possible exercise.
> Habituate yourself to walk very fast."
> **Thomas Jefferson**

Walking is an especially easy activity to squeeze into our day. We can take a walk during our break times or lunch period at work. Some of our meetings can be done while walking. We can walk while we talk on the phone. We can get off the bus a stop or two early and walk the extra distance. We can walk while waiting to catch a flight. There are many good reasons why walking is the most popular aerobic exercise and has the lowest dropout rate.

Running is also enormously popular and for good reason. Even if you've never enjoyed it in the past, you might want to consider trying it again. It has an addictive quality that is priceless once achieved. Ask any runner how they felt about running when they first started. You'll find few people enjoyed running from the outset even though they love it now. Even Tom Holland, endurance athlete and author of *The Marathon Method*, is quick to admit he found his three-mile runs to be horrible in the beginning.

Like most people, I also used to dislike running. It seemed to me that only a masochist could enjoy it. Then in my senior year of college, a friend told me that if I stuck with it for six weeks I would be addicted and unable to stop. The next year I decided to give her advice a try. Six weeks of running came and went and it would have been quite easy for me to quit. Fortunately, I chose to stick with it. After six months it finally happened; at that point you couldn't have paid me to quit. This may seem like an awfully long time to have pushed myself to stay with it, but running has been an important fixture in maintaining my fitness ever since. Clearly, this six-month investment has yielded immeasurable returns.

Lifestyle Fitness

It was previously generally believed that exercising for durations of less than 30 minutes provided very little benefit. More recent research, though, has found that three 10-minute exercise sessions are just as effective as one 30-minute session. This is fantastic news for those looking to spread movement throughout their day. Household chores can even become part of our fitness program. For example, you could achieve the minimum recommended level of activity for a day with 10 minutes of raking, 10 minutes of mopping, and a 10-minute walk to the store.

Spend some time looking for ways to integrate more activity into your existing lifestyle. Is there somewhere you go regularly where you could ride your bike instead of using your car? How about always parking in the farthest parking spot from the store or office front door? You'll simplify what can easily become a time-consuming battle for the closest spot and furthermore, consider the door dings you'll avoid. These types of small changes are often easier to adopt than grand-scale efforts.

With the plethora of wearable activity trackers now available, many people target taking a certain number of steps in a day. Having a goal of achieving 10,000 steps has become common. This approach allows tremendous flexibility because it can be done in so many ways.

Consider activities that would save you money or provide some other type of value. Wash your own car. Mow your own grass. Just because there are options to accomplish things with less effort doesn't mean these are the best choices when considering our bodies' need to be used.

Seasonal Changes

Being unprepared for the change in seasons frequently puts an end to people's exercise routine. It may be the off-season for our chosen sport, the weather may no longer be well suited to what we have been doing, or there may be a lack of sufficient daylight. Despite knowing the change is coming, many fail to plan for it. Be one of those who are prepared.

You change throughout the year, just as Mother Nature does. Do you prefer a big hearty stew more on a hot summer's day or in the dead of winter? It's natural—although not required—to be less active in the winter months. While it's important to keep exercising, it's reasonable to expect a decline in activity level. Have a plan to keep the shorter days and stormy weather from breaking your exercise habit and causing you to drop below your minimum acceptable activity level.

I'm sure you've heard the saying, "Variety is the spice of life." Changing your activities with the change of the seasons keeps you from becoming bored with them. Doing the exact same routine each week, month, and year eventually leads to burnout. Even professional athletes change the type and focus of their training throughout the year.

Establish a variety of possibilities that include both indoor and outdoor activities you enjoy. A seasonal approach may look something like this:

Season	Outdoor Activity	Indoor Activity
Spring	Hiking, Soccer	Circuit training
Summer	Swimming, Cycling	Racquetball
Fall	Jogging, Softball	Volleyball
Winter	Skiing, Snowshoeing	Dancing

Even if your seasonal changes are minimal, some amount of variation is needed to stay mentally fresh. Also, your body will be better balanced when you do a variety of activities. Just as eating a variety of foods is best for optimum health, so is engaging in a variety of physical activities. A seasonal approach is healthier and more natural.

How Much

To determine the amount of exercise you should do, you need to again consider what you are trying to achieve. Are you more concerned with weight loss or generally improving your health?

For the purpose of weight loss, you can determine the amount of exercise you need based on your weight loss goals. You can find the caloric burn for many different activities at a number of different Internet sites. Knowing the rate at which an activity burns calories allows you to then calculate how much of it you need to do to reach your goals.

Let's assume Beth wants to lose a pound per week through a combination of diet and exercise. A pound of fat contains roughly 3,200 calories. She has decided she will forgo her daily 300-calorie latte. Skipping the coffee will account for a reduction of 2,100 (7 x 300) calories per week. This leaves 1,100 (3,200 – 2,100) calories a week to be burned through exercise in order to reach her goal.

Beth has decided to jog for exercise. Jogging burns roughly 100 calories per mile. From this burn rate, we can easily calculate that she will need to jog 11 miles a week to get the result she is after.

Determining the amount of exercise required to improve overall health of the body is more difficult. Researchers have been working for decades to determine the answer. A task force of government and private concerns joined together to create a report titled *2008 Physical Activity Guidelines for Americans* which, according to the U.S. Department of Health & Human Services, represents the first comprehensive guidelines on physical activity ever issued by the federal government. It's still widely accepted as the standard.

The following recommendations are based on its guidelines.

Cardiovascular Training

It is recommended that adults between the ages of 18 and 64 engage in a minimum of 150 minutes of moderate-intensity aerobic activity each week. If vigorous-intensity aerobic activity is done, the time required is cut in half to 75 minutes.

These guidelines are consistent with those previously published by the American College of Sports Medicine and the American Heart Association, which recommend people engage in at least 30 minutes of moderate-intensity physical activity five days per week.

There are additional health benefits from doing more than the recommended minimum level, but there is also a point of diminishing returns. Research suggests that doing twice the recommended minimum will continue to produce measurable health improvements.

Moderate-intensity aerobic activity produces a heart rate from 60% to 74% of the person's maximum heart rate. Vigorous intensity is working at 75% to 85% of maximum heart rate. To determine what percentage of maximum heart rate you're using, you'll need to know your current heart rate and maximum heart rate.

Maximum heart rate varies from person to person. There are tests that can be done to establish a person's maximum heart rate, but most use the simple equation of 220 beats per minute (BPM) minus the person's age as a good rule of thumb. Using this formula, a 40-year-old person has a maximum heart rate of 180 BPM (220 − 40).

Determining current heart rate can be done by taking your pulse and counting the number of beats in a minute (or count for 30 seconds and multiply by two or count for 15 seconds and multiple by four). While this method is easy and reliable, an even better method is to buy a heart rate monitor. The cost of heart rate monitors has dropped substantially over the years; a monitor may now be purchased for less than $15. It's a worthwhile investment to have a continuous reading of your heart rate. Also, there is additional useful information they can provide. For example, some will record your activity level all day long and calculate total calories burned for the day.

Having both the current and maximum heart rates, we can calculate the percentage of maximum we are operating at. As an example, assume a 50-year-old man has a heart rate of 119 BPM. His maximum heart rate is 170 (220 − 50). He is working at 70% of his maximum rate (119 / 170), and therefore, at a moderate-intensity aerobic level.

If measuring your intensity through heart rate doesn't appeal to you, there is another option. You can use the "talk test," which focuses on breathing rate rather than heart rate. Moderate intensity is when a person can hold a conversation, but would be short of breath trying to sing. Vigorous intensity is when only a few words can be said between breaths. Your intensity is too great if you are desperate to stop or it makes you feel as though you want to avoid exercise.

Strength Training

It's recommended that, in addition to aerobic exercise, people do strength training two or more days of the week. Ideally, this should work all of the major muscle groups, including the chest, shoulders, stomach, back, hips, legs, and arms.

No specific amount of time is recommended. The guidance is to do between one to three sets of 8 to 12 repetitions when doing resistance training. The muscles should be taxed to the point that doing one more repetition would be difficult without help.

Flexibility Training

There are currently no minimum levels of flexibility training recommended by the report. Yet it remains important because flexibility training is what allows you to do the other two types of exercise over the long haul, as it counteracts the continuous shortening of your muscles that they cause. Since shortening of the muscles can easily contribute to injury, flexibility training provides preventative maintenance for your exercise program.

Stretching can be easier to integrate into your life than the other two forms of exercise. You can attend classes that focus on stretching, such as yoga, but if you'd like to attend another type of fitness classes, it'll usually already include a segment dedicated to stretching. When doing an aerobic activity, it's often used as part of a warm up, cool down, or both. You can also easily establish your own home routine, which can be dispersed throughout your day at your convenience, often even while doing other things. For example, you can stretch while talking on the telephone, watching television, reading, or while you're waiting for something, like your computer to boot or a pot of water to boil. You may also enjoy combining your stretching with a few moments of silence and deep breathing, which can provide rejuvenation for your body and spirit throughout the day.

Intelligent Progression

Exercise is an evolutionary process. The amount, intensity, type, and setting will change over time just as all of the other facets of your life eventually change. The human body likes consistency, though, so it's best if changes in activity levels are gradual. It's truly amazing what the body will adapt to, but it needs time to adjust.

Caution in the amount of exercise you do is more important in the beginning than at any other time. Almost without exception, people try to do too much, too soon. If you're in it for the long haul, there is no need to rush things. In fact, rushing things will only hinder you. Doing too much may cause an injury. Worse yet, overexertion can cause you to associate exercise with pain.

> "It is the direction and not the magnitude which is to be taken into consideration."
>
> **Thomas Paine**

The government report mentioned in the previous section states, "In general, healthy men and women who plan prudent increases in their weekly amounts of physical activity do not need to consult a health-care provider before becoming active." If you haven't been active for quite some time or have disabilities or health issues, it would be wise to get your doctor's input on your exercise plan.

Frequency, duration, and intensity all need to be carefully controlled. Studies have shown that exercise dropout rates are higher for those who increase intensity and duration quickly. If you haven't been doing any exercise, start by exercising just once or twice a week for the first couple of weeks. Increase the frequency when you're ready, but don't step up by more than one day per week each time you are prepared to do more.

When deciding how long to exercise in a single session, start with a duration you can complete without too much exertion, based on your current level of conditioning. Increase exercise time in increments in the 10% to 20% range. As mentioned earlier, three 10-minute bouts of exercise during a day are just as beneficial as a single 30-minute session. Use this to your advantage in the beginning by doing short workouts and allowing your endurance to build up gradually. Judge your success on the progress you make rather than how you compare to others.

You can gradually work toward having one workout per week that's more difficult than the others. This serves to make most workouts feel relatively easy. For example, if John runs four times per week, three miles each time, all of his workouts are equally difficult. If he replaces one of his three-mile runs with a weekly four-mile run, he will find that three out of his four workouts for the week seem relatively easy. It's worth it to work a little harder one day a week so that the rest of the week seems easier.

Start at the lower range of the moderate intensity level (60% to 70% of maximum heart rate). Many are surprised how relatively comfortable they are exercising at this level. Having in the past adhered to the old "no pain, no gain" adage, they pushed themselves to the point of gasping for air with muscles screaming. They feel a little guilty going at an easy pace, as though exercise was meant to be some sort of punishment. But it's not. Learn proper intensity and your body with thank you.

Don't increase intensity while exercise frequency and duration are being increased. Intensity is the last of the three elements to be increased, if you decide to increase it at all.

This may seem to some to be a conservative progression, but I have yet to see someone stop exercising because of starting off too gradually. Droves stop because of starting off too fast. Remember that there are more adaptations required beyond those your body will be making. Your mental attitude, schedule, habits, and friends and family need to adjust, as well. They'll adjust more easily given sufficient time to adapt.

Many want to dive in and go all out to capitalize on their newfound motivation to exercise. Try to avoid this type of thinking. The idea that we must seize a limited-time opportunity plants the idea in your head that exercise will be a short-lived endeavor. Instead, channel any extra motivation you feel into developing a solid exercise plan and effective long-term strategy to incorporate exercise as an ongoing part of your lifestyle. If you have spent years getting out of shape, it doesn't make much sense to try to get back into shape in just a few short weeks. Give the process time and put some thought into it.

Now that we've covered the exercise basics, you can begin to develop an exercise plan. The following chapter will guide you through how to develop your own personalized plan that meshes nicely with you and your lifestyle. With this plan in hand, you'll be on your way to long-term success.

CHAPTER HIGHLIGHTS

Types of Exercise
- Aerobic, strengthening, and flexibility exercises each provide different benefits.

Activity Selection
- Be creative yet practical in identifying a variety of activities you'll enjoy.

How Much
- Work up to at least 150 minutes a week of moderate intensity aerobic exercise, balanced with some strength and flexibility training.

Intelligent Progression
- Make gradual changes to your activity levels

ACTION STEPS

✔ Find a new activity or class to try.

✔ Identify the easiest way you could fit in some walking or jogging.

✔ Outline a seasonal approach.

✔ Invest in a heart rate monitor.

Chapter 7

Create Your Plan

"It takes as much energy to wish as it does to plan."

Eleanor Roosevelt

Goals

As the electronic age has made it easier to connect with other people, organizations, information, and entertainment, the number of people and things calling for our attention has risen dramatically. Many fail to stick with their exercise program because they lose focus; to prevent this outcome, you need a system that will keep your desire to be fit from becoming lost in a sea of distractions. Good intentions don't equal good results without a good plan.

Some people subconsciously avoid creating a plan because if we have no plan, we cannot fail. Equally true, however, is if we have no plan, we cannot succeed. Have you ever noticed you instantly feel better once you have developed a plan to solve a dilemma? We inherently know that having a plan is a critical first step in moving from floundering to progressing. It provides relief for the pain of feeling like we are going nowhere.

> "Definitiveness of purpose is the starting point of all achievement."
>
> **W. Clement Stone**

The starting point for a good plan is to establish goals. Undoubtedly, you have repeatedly heard of the importance of goal setting. This is because nothing is more important in guiding us to a result we want than defining what that result is. Look back at your more significant achievements in life and you'll find most of them resulted from having had a goal. Worthwhile achievements rarely happen accidentally.

Well-defined, concrete goals are needed. For the best results, create SMART goals, an acronym commonly defined as follows:

S = Specific

M = Measurable

A = Action oriented

R = Realistic

T = Time bound

Specific

Vague goals such as "I'm going to exercise more" produce ambiguous results. You need to know exactly what it is you want to achieve. An example of a specific goal would be to walk for 30 minutes every other day.

Measurable

You need the ability to determine if you are succeeding or failing. This requires your goals to be measurable in some way in order to gauge your progress. Time and frequency, like used in the previous example, are good measures. Distance can also be used, such as a goal to walk three miles, three times a week.

Action Oriented

In Chapter 4, you identified the outcomes you wish to achieve through exercise. Since these are the reasons you have decided to exercise, it may seem only logical these would be your exercise goals. The problem with using these outcomes as your goals is that, while exercise will produce positive results, the rate and ultimate achievement is affected by many other factors beyond exercise itself. Here are a couple examples to illustrate.

Imagine someone who began exercising to lose weight simultaneously started a daily habit of eating banana splits. If that person didn't lose any weight, would it make sense for him or her to quit exercising because the goal of losing weight was not achieved? Obviously, the answer is no. Exercise made a positive contribution by burning additional calories, even though the stated goal wasn't met. Without exercise, weight would have been gained.

Consider a person that decided to use exercise to reduce stress and began exercising about the time his or her mother-in-law moved in. The adjustment to having a new household member was difficult. Privacy and space were lost, while demands and drama increased. In this environment, the person's stress might actually increase rather than go down. Again, the outcome-related goal of stress reduction wasn't achieved, although exercise made a positive contribution. Dealing with the situation would have been more difficult without the stress relief exercise provided.

Another problem with outcome-based goals is that it's hard to know how quickly we'll obtain certain results. Each of our bodies is a little different. For example, two people with varying metabolic rates and percentages of lean muscle could follow an identical fitness routine and get distinctly different results. There are many variables in play, which makes it difficult to predict the timing of results.

Almost universally, people overestimate how quickly they'll see results. And our society is increasingly feeding our expectation of instant results. Then when the changes don't come as quickly as we had expected, we become discouraged. In this way, outcome-based goals can easily end up serving as a de-motivator if used as the basis for setting goals. Our desire for the results exercise will bring is vital, but its importance is in keeping us committed to sticking with our exercise plan, not in creating it.

The purpose of your goals is to allow you to formulate a good plan. Your goals need to focus on the activity of exercise: the types of activities you'll do, how frequently, for how long and how intensely. Consistently following an intelligent plan will eventually lead to the results you want.

Realistic

Optimism is a favorable trait; however, in goal setting, it can lead you to overcommit and set yourself up for failure. I have often seen people who haven't been exercising at all set a goal to start exercising every day. I've yet to see one of these people succeed. It's discouraging when we always come up short of our goals. On the other hand, it's satisfying when you achieve your goals and invigorating when you exceed them. Set your goals at a level where this can happen.

Time Bound

Without the parameters of time, you aren't setting goals, you are merely dreaming. Things you are going to accomplish "someday" have no power to create action. Things that lack enough importance to have a deadline lack enough importance to ever get done. Cleaning that junk drawer in your home lacks the importance of a deadline and will, therefore, forever remain a junk drawer. Use time commitments to save your exercise plans from the fate of becoming part of your mental junk drawer—things you'll do someday "when you have time."

If exercise is to be part of your daily life, you need both short-term and long-term goals. You need short-term goals that direct what you'll do this week. You need long-term goals to guide how your weekly goals change over time.

For example, you could have a long-term goal of running a 1/2 marathon race (13.1 miles) within the next two years. If you're not presently running at all, your initial short-term weekly goal might be to walk for 20 minutes three times with one minute of slow jogging in the middle. In future weeks, you would gradually increase the time spent jogging and reduce the amount of time spent walking. After getting up to running for the full 20 minutes, you would start making the workout a little longer. These would be SMART goals with your weekly goal moving you toward your long-term goal.

Create long-term goals that will provide a sense of pride and accomplishment. For example, you could set a goal to accumulate the number of miles walking, jogging, or cycling that would allow you to cross the state you live in. If stair climbing is part of your fitness, you could set a long-term goal of logging the number of steps you'd need to climb the 29,028-foot elevation of Mt. Everest. The more tangible and meaningful the goal feels, the better it is.

Setting a goal and maintaining a consistent focus on it creates a natural pull toward it. You'll start to notice and realize things that help you achieve it. You'll find opportunities you didn't see before. Nothing is more powerful in creating a result than a consistent focus on your goals.

Scheduling

Common sense tells us that if we are going to engage in moderate intensity aerobic activity for the recommended 150 minutes per week, 30 minutes five times a week would be better for us than once a week for two and a half hours. When pursuing fitness goals, the "weekend warrior" approach is best avoided. Spread exercise throughout the week as evenly as possible.

The time you plan to spend exercising will most often need to be scheduled. There may be days when you spontaneously decide to do some sort of physical activity; however, few people have enough of these inspired moments to provide the body with sufficient exercise. In other words, it won't work to just exercise when you feel like it.

Most long-term exercisers have a standard routine they follow. For some it's a daily regime, while others operate from a standard weekly schedule. In any case, they know in advance when they'll exercise. If you want something to happen, you must plan a time for it.

> "The key is not to prioritize what's on your schedule, but to schedule your priorities."
>
> **Stephen Covey**

Selecting a time to exercise is where many go wrong. A common approach is to reserve time for all of life's other commitments and then choose a time to exercise based on any leftover time slots. If we truly want the benefits exercise has to offer and recognize its importance as a part of our lifestyle, why would it be last on the list in scheduling? If it really is a priority in our lives, it needs to be scheduled that way.

Deciding when you'll exercise is critical to success. The need for sufficient energy to overcome the law of inertia and to fortify willpower was discussed in Chapter 2. With this in mind, you need to consider your typical energy levels when deciding when you'll exercise.

Daily Rhythms

Our energy level naturally fluctuates throughout the day. Humans, like most living things, are impacted by what is known as circadian rhythms. Each of us has biologically programmed daily highs and lows in our energy level. Humans possess internal time clocks that change the production level of certain hormones and proteins throughout the day, which impact our alertness and energy. Although humans tend to have similar patterns, such as being less alert and sleepier mid-afternoon and at night, they are not identical. We each have unique genetics that impact our cycle. For example, you may be or know a "night owl," someone who is most alert and productive at night.

You may already know your normal daily energy pattern. If not, take the time to chart your energy level for a few days and you'll quickly see a pattern develop. Let's use the pattern an aspiring triathlete, Hector, discovered as an example.

In the below chart, 10 represents peak energy.

Normal Daily Energy Cycle

Level	5AM	6AM	7AM	8AM	9AM	10AM	11AM	12PM	1PM	2PM	3PM	4PM	5PM	6PM	7PM	8PM	9PM	10PM
10				x	x													
9																		
8			x			x		x										
7							x		x	x								
6														x	x			
5												x	x					
4											x					x		
3																	x	
2		x																x
1	x																	

The charting helped Hector see why he was finding it difficult to roll out of bed and do a workout before work. After identifying his energy patterns, he was able to rearrange his work schedule to start a little later on Tuesdays and Thursdays, which let him wait until 7 a.m. to start his workout. This has made it much easier for him to get in a morning workout on those days. Targeting weekend workouts for 8 a.m. or 9 a.m. has worked extremely well since this is his peak energy period. On Mondays, Wednesdays, and Fridays, he does a lunchtime workout instead of a morning workout. In addition, he tries to leave a little early for his lunchtime workout, knowing his energy level will be slightly higher then. He has enough energy to do early evening workouts, but since he knows he will have to push himself harder to get going, he chooses to instead schedule activity earlier in the day.

Time of Day

It's important to face the reality that the later in the day you schedule exercise, the lower the odds are that you'll do it. The chances of something interfering are greater, and there is less opportunity to utilize a backup plan. This is not to say that a plan to exercise in the evenings is doomed to fail. Many people successfully work activity in, enjoying how it provides a buffer between their work life and home life. According to the U.S. Bureau of Labor Statistics, 6 p.m. is the most common time working people exercise during the workweek. It is, however, still important to consider the pitfalls.

Many people don't consider the options of altering their standard 8-5 workday to fit in exercise. Certainly there are many cases where altering a work schedule is not practical; however, don't be too hasty in deciding you don't have this ability. Just because nobody else in the organization is doing it doesn't mean it won't be allowed.

Intelligent companies and bosses know the value of fit and healthy employees. Fit employees have lower costs and produce more work than unfit employees. This is why many companies have invested money to create fit workforces. They have built gyms for their employees, contributed to health club memberships, or provided other incentives. As a result, they have seen reductions in healthcare costs, absenteeism, and disability leaves while simultaneously seeing improvements in productivity and morale.

In 2007, the American Heart Association reported that the average company can expect a benefit of $3.40 to $7.88 for every $1 it spends on a worksite wellness program. More recent studies from various organizations have also found results within this range. Allowing flexibility in start times or lunch periods are a small price for a company to pay for the added productivity, reduced absenteeism, and reduced healthcare costs that result. Some companies have gone so far as to allow employees to use work time to exercise and found that these employees maintained the same work output, or higher, despite spending less time on the job.

While it has typically been larger companies that have invested in fitness and wellness programs, the benefits are the same for smaller companies. In fact, the importance is arguably greater for smaller companies, where each employee has a bigger impact on the company's bottom line results and the need to control costs is even more critical.

You're doing your employer a big favor by becoming fit, and you shouldn't hesitate to ask for support. It may seem that you are a better employee by working through your lunch rather than going off to exercise, but the opposite is actually true. Studies have shown employees who take a midday break, especially if it's to exercise, are more productive than those who attempt to "power through." The best employees take care of their health and maintain a high energy level and positive outlook. Chances are actually good that your company will appreciate the example you set.

Exercise doesn't always have to entail working up a sweat. To avoid the need for a shower during the workday, you can do short bouts of activity. As mentioned early, just 10 minutes of exercise can make a measurable contribution to fitness. You can also do non-aerobic activities. Pilates, yoga, or tai chi all have the potential to improve your body without the need to sweat.

Weekly Plans

Fine tune your exercise plan on a weekly basis. Consider the upcoming special events, celebrations, travel, appointments, or other commitments that you may need to adjust for. Check the weather forecasts. Consider what's likely to not go according to plan. You can often predict situations that may detour your exercise plans. Obstacles are easier to overcome when you have anticipated them and are already prepared.

> "By failing to prepare you are preparing to fail."
> **Benjamin Franklin**

Also within your weekly plan, consider the chores and activities you intend to do during the week. Will you be tilling the garden or helping a friend move? These activities count as exercise even though they're not done just for the sake of exercise.

Communicate your plan to your support team (as established in Chapter 5). This allows them to be prepared to provide the support you may need. They'll be able to determine what accommodations they need to make and when they may need to provide encouragement.

When scheduling, note which of the PREP conditions (pleasure, routine, energy, and people) will exist for each workout. If there are days when it will be just one of the four conditions, see if you can come up with a way to get it to two. The more of them present, the better the chances are you'll follow through.

Record your exercise plan for the week. Enter it into whatever tool you use to record your other appointments: the calendar on your wall, your computer, or your phone. This will help you avoid missing workouts by simply forgetting. This appointment with yourself is as important as any other on your schedule, so needs to be treated in the same way.

> "Stay committed to your decisions,
> but stay flexible in your approach."
> **Tony Robbins**

Having an established workout backup plan helps consistency. If your plan to exercise in the morning or midday is foiled, know how you'll change your normal evening routine to fit in a workout. Know the specifics of what the activity will be, what you'll skip that evening to make time for it, and how you'll raise your energy level enough to get started.

The hard truth is sometimes the barriers to exercise are going to win. An interference will come up you couldn't have anticipated. This is why it's important to establish make-up days in your schedule. Making fitness part of your lifestyle is easier if there is some flexibility. Although exercising consistently is important, it's not necessary that you exercise every day of your life. You needn't feel bad about missing a scheduled workout one day if you make up for it on another. No harm, no foul. If you miss on your make-up day, *then* it's time to take a hard look at what's going on around you and inside of you.

Using Experience

Likely you have heard it said that experience is the best teacher. Frequently people don't take advantage of this truism when it comes to exercise. They assume past failures were simply from a lack of resolve and they just need to try harder this time.

Failed attempts provide a fertile learning opportunity. Take the time to analyze your past attempts to exercise regularly and identify both things that helped and those that got in the way. Start by recalling your exercise experience and concentrate on those things that made it better or you found helpful. Use the following questions to jog your memory:

- What did you enjoy about the activity?

- What things did you try that made it even better?

- Who was supportive?

- What helped you fit it into your schedule?

- What motivated you?

Also analyze what caused you to stop. Go beyond the first reason that comes to mind. Reasons like "I wasn't motivated enough to keep going" or "I got too busy" don't provide sufficient information for you to know what to do differently this time. Use the following questions to dig deeper and find specific, actionable information:

- What was your typical energy level at the time you were supposed to start to exercise?

- What were you focusing on during the workouts and how did you feel?

- What things did you dislike about the activity?

- What things happened that are likely to happen again?

- Did you try to do too much, too soon, causing burnout or injury?

- What were your repetitive negative thoughts?

- What conflicts arose?

- What was inconvenient?

- What was the impact of your old habits?

- Is there a common thread or pattern from each time you stopped exercising?

> "The successful man will profit from his mistakes
> and try again in a different way."
>
> **Dale Carnegie**

Your answers to these questions will indicate what you need to repeat and what you need to change in your approach. Did the time of day, type of activity, or plan design create problems or was it your mental attitude? Knowing the specifics allows the issues to be addressed.

Habit Development

As briefly discussed in Chapter 2, humans are creatures of habit. Most of what we say, think, and do is out of habit. As much as most of us like to think of ourselves as free and unbridled, the truth is we spend most of our time in the well-worn trenches of habit. This is why it's critical that exercise develops into a habit. It won't survive as part of your life any other way.

> "It's not what we do once in a while that shapes our lives,
> but what we do consistently."
>
> **Tony Robbins**

It's important to recognize the powerful influences your habits create. Essentially, you are your habits. The more you do something, the more natural it becomes and the more it becomes part of who you are. Habits direct how you live your life. What you do in a typical day is based on habit and what you do in a typical day predominately determines what you'll accomplish and experience in life. In a very real way, your habits determine the quality of your life and the person you are.

We can't get away from having habits; they are essential for functioning in today's world. Habits reduce the time and energy required for analysis and decision making. We couldn't function if we had to consider millions of options in what to think, say, and do every moment of every day. We would soon go mad.

Like thoughts, habits aren't inherently positive or negative. *Choices* determine their nature. Everyone has both good and bad habits. The underpinning to all self-improvement is in improving our habits, particularly replacing bad habits with good ones.

> "Men acquire a particular quality
> by constantly acting in a particular way."
> **Aristotle**

Evaluate your current habits to determine how they will affect your intentions to exercise. Pay special attention to the routines you currently follow leading up to the time you plan to use for exercise. Identify those that will interfere with your exercise plan.

For example, my friend Robyn told me she had decided to start jogging in the mornings before work. She was going to make a habit of getting up at 5:30 a.m. instead of her usual

6:15 a.m. I commended her and asked if she was going to also make it a habit of going to bed 45 minutes earlier than she does now.

It hadn't yet occurred to her that she had more than one habit to change. I pointed out that if she started getting less sleep, her morning fatigue would eventually override her motivation for her morning jog. She was able to recognize this was likely to happen and thought about her normal evening routine. She usually likes to check email and social media later in the evening just before going to bed. Since she didn't want to give this up, she had more habits to change in order to fit this in earlier in the evening.

It's important to recognize the domino effect of your habits. Robyn probably wouldn't have been successful in exercising before work for long if she hadn't first identified the implications of her other habits and adjusted them as necessary. Identify each one of your habits that needs to be changed to support your new exercise habit.

Habitual Thinking

Our habits are more than the routines we follow throughout the day. We have habits in what we think and say. When greeting others, we tend to have a habitual response, such as "Hi, how are you?" or "It's nice to meet you." We rely on these mental and verbal habits each day just as much as we do our physical habits.

Establishing an exercise habit goes beyond simply creating physical routines. Creating supportive mental and verbal habits are equally important.

> "Motivation is what gets you started.
> Habit is what keeps you going."
> **Jim Ryan**

What do you normally think about before a workout? Do you think about how good you'll feel when you're done, or do you think about how sluggish you feel at this moment? What do you say to people before heading out for a workout? It should be easy to determine which of these patterns support your exercise habit and which don't. Replace any habitual self-defeating thoughts with your personal exercise slogan developed from Chapter 4.

Unfortunately, your habitual patterns of thinking and doing may be deeply ingrained. You have probably heard the saying, "Old habits die hard." The longer they have been with you, the harder they'll be to change. Also, the more habits you need to change, the more challenge you should expect.

> "Could the young but realize how soon they will become
> mere walking bundles of habits, they would give more heed
> to their conduct while in the plastic state."
> **William James**

Part of the difficulty in changing habits is their stealth nature. We fall into our habitual patterns without even realizing it. After repeating a pattern for long enough, our brain creates a neurological script it activates when the correct stimulus triggers it. This script becomes part of our wiring, which is why we can perform habitual activities without thinking. The problem is that when we change our goals, this ingrained script doesn't simply vanish. Findings from research on habit have found that it's frequently not a lack of willpower or understanding of health issues that keep people from exercising. Their findings suggest it's the power of situations to trigger past habits that often override the best of intentions.

We can change our habits, but it may require considerable focus and effort. Pay close attention to the triggers for your habits that interfere with exercise. The trigger can be the time of day, a location, something someone says, or other habits. It's in recognizing these triggers that you are able to use your awareness to make a conscious choice and avoid the interfering habit.

Since one habit can trigger another, you'll develop an exercise habit more easily if you attach it to an existing habit. Look at your current habits and find one you can hitch your new exercise habit to.

Reward System

It's human nature to desire instant gratification. Marketers play upon this desire and our society caters to it. Most of us now demand and expect instant gratification in virtually all aspects of our daily lives. Luckily, exercise is capable of delivering immediate gratification, and you should look for the positive results from each workout.

Unfortunately, it can take time to condition ourselves to focus on the positive aspects. Also, many of the benefits and positive associations of exercise develop gradually and aren't easily recognized in the beginning. Yet this is precisely the time we most need to see the benefits to improve our chances of creating exercise as a habit.

For this reason, it can be helpful to develop a reward system you can use until exercise becomes habit and its own reward. The rate in which people get to this state varies tremendously, but you'll know when you've arrived. In the meanwhile, determining some rewards can be helpful.

There are different approaches you can take. You could set a small reward for each workout you do or a big reward after completing a certain number of them. Some of the rewards I've seen used are clothes, shoes, music, movies, massage, a weekend getaway, and a trip to Hawaii. Rewards become powerful motivators based on their magnitude, certainty, and immediacy. So choose something you'll truly look forward to and make sure to follow through as soon as it's earned.

Rewards do more than treat us to something we want; they also create an acknowledgement of our success. For many of us, this positive mental boost is the real value. Why do I put the blue ribbon I won on my wall or a trophy on my mantel? These things serve no useful purpose—except to remind me of my accomplishments. Acknowledge the importance of exercise by rewarding yourself for it.

Using what you have learned so far, you should be ready to create a highly personalized exercise plan. Think about it, write it down, and share it with your support team. In the next chapter, you'll learn techniques that will help you stick with your plan.

CHAPTER HIGHLIGHTS

Goals
- A fitness plan starts with clearly defined goals.

Scheduling
- Successful scheduling requires exercise be given sufficient priority and timed to coincide with higher energy states.

Using Experience
- The most effective personal approaches to exercise are guided by the lessons of past experiences.

Habit Development
- Exercise must develop into a habit to remain part of your life.

Reward System
- Rewards can add motivation until exercise becomes its own reward.

ACTION STEPS

✔ Develop SMART exercise goals.

✔ Identify your energy patterns.

✔ Establish the tools you will use to schedule exercise on a weekly basis.

✔ Identify what can be learned from past exercise experiences.

✔ Identify any habits you have that could interfere with exercise.

✔ Create rewards for achieving exercise goals.

✔ Create a written exercise plan utilizing all of the above information and the action steps from previous chapters. Share this with your support team and review it often.

Chapter 8

Sticking with It

"Energy and persistence conquer all things."

Benjamin Franklin

Tracking Results

In the previous chapter, you determined your specific goals in order to clearly target what you want. The next step is to take action and record your results. We all recognize we need to take action to get the results we want. What many fail to recognize, however, is the importance of recording those actions.

The need for accountability was discussed in Chapter 4. Without accountability, our good intentions are often swept away as easily as feathers in the wind. You create accountability by measuring progress and results. I suggest you maintain a log to compare the workouts you completed to those you had planned. This is especially important before exercise has developed into a habit.

Maintaining a log requires only a few minutes a week, a small investment especially when you consider the benefits it provides. An exercise log:

- Provides measurement of results, which allows objective judgment of progress (accountability)

- Promotes clarity of goals

- Helps maintain focus

- Provides valuable historical information

Consider expanding what you record to also include the following:

- Your feelings about the workout

- Anything special that happened

- Things that obstructed your workout

- Aches and pains

- Logistical items, such as, time, place, and weather

Recording this extra information will shed light on why you received the results you did; expose patterns, either good or bad; encourage learning and discovery; help you avoid injury by keeping you attuned to warning signs; and help you build an emotional connection and deep commitment to exercise.

> "However beautiful the strategy,
> you should occasionally look at the results."
> **Winston Churchill**

Another benefit produced by tracking results is that it fosters a sense of accomplishment. All too often in life, we don't take the time to recognize and appreciate our achievements. While maintaining your fitness log, be sure to take notice of what you have achieved. It feels good to take pride in your successes, and your log provides the opportunity to reflect on your achievements. Even if you didn't accomplish all that you set out to do, you'll be reminded of the activities you did do—every completed workout is something to be proud of. Take the time to pat yourself on the back for the obstacles you overcame to make each of them happen. Acknowledge your success and carry the positive energy of your accomplishments into the next week.

There are plenty of options when it comes to logs. You can find free logs to download on the Internet, create an online account at a website that offers tracking, buy a log book or journal, or create your own.

There has been an explosion in the use of "wearables," watch-like tracking devices worn on the wrist. These devices record your activity and transfer the data to your smartphone. Through a phone application, the data is also transferred to the Internet for viewing online. While worn, the wearable continuously tracks your activities, recording how much walking, running, cycling, etc., is done. Heart rate and calories burned are also tracked and displayed, and some models even record the amount and quality of sleep you receive.

Wearables provide continuous, real-time feedback on your activity level and also include associated online programs that can provide support in other areas, such as recommendations for improvement, goal setting, and social support. They're certainly the most expensive option, but you may find the investment well worth it.

Whatever method you use, you can increase the motivational power of your workout log by posting it where others will see it. If it's an online log, you can allow others to view it. If you're using a paper log, put it on your refrigerator or somewhere visible in your workspace. It fortifies our motivation when we know others will see what we have (or have not) accomplished.

If maintaining a log seems like too much trouble and you're not interested in or able to purchase a wearable, at the very least record your time spent exercising on a wall calendar. It only takes a few moments and, although it won't provide the full benefits of a log, will allow you to hold yourself accountable.

Conquering Challenges

Things may start off perfectly, but sooner or later you're bound to run into challenges. Other demands will get in the way or you may start accepting flimsy excuses to not exercise. This is where exercise ends for most.

Recognize that the obstacles you face are problems to be solved, not simply reasons to quit. These obstacles can, in fact, be great opportunities: our failures often teach us more than our successes and overcoming challenges is how we grow and improve. Furthermore, it turns out that our chances of success are improved if we have failed in the past and learned from the attempt.

For these reasons, it's nearly as valuable to record what kept you from doing a workout as it is to record a workout you completed. When recording missed workouts, you should note a number of factors: the major reason you missed your workout, what you were thinking about and feeling at the time, and who, if anyone, influenced you. This gives you concrete information you can use in solving the problem. It also keeps you from going for days without stopping to question why you've gotten off track.

> "Success consists of going from failure to failure without loss of enthusiasm."
>
> **Winston Churchill**

When reviewing this information, look for patterns to see if you can identify a deeper reason than the one you recorded. For example, if you stopped going to the gym because your dog ate your membership card, realize there is more to it than that. Examine your feelings to pinpoint the exact problem. Different problems require different solutions, so get clear on the real issue. Make sure you are treating the illness rather than the symptoms. Do you have feelings of frustration, guilt, or exhaustion? What is making you feel this way? Are these feelings coming from something you are telling yourself or from what others are saying to you?

Once you understand the root of the problem, shift to solving it. Your first idea may not be your best. Take the time to identify at least three possible solutions. Identify three pros and three cons for each potential solution. Be creative. Rely on your support network for ideas. The more options you have to choose from the more likely you'll find the perfect solution.

Sometimes missed workouts are simply the result of insufficient forethought and organization. Take note of when missing a workout could have been avoided with better planning. Do you sometimes forget your gym bag? Is there a meeting that often runs late and interferes with your exercise plan? Develop strategies to be better prepared. Have a backup plan. Do you need to leave a spare set of gym clothes in the trunk of your car or at the office? Could you develop a strategy of how to gracefully exit the meeting when it runs late? Is there a different workout you could do later at home?

If you're not missing workouts, but find yourself dreading them, recognize this as a sign that a change is needed. Notice what aspect of it you are focusing on. Likely, you're anticipating you're going to be uncomfortable before you even begin. It's natural to want to avoid discomfort, so it's critical that this anticipation be dealt with. As much as I appreciate the benefits of exercise, I would fail to stick with it if I thought I was going to be miserable throughout each workout. To address this negative mindset, there are three things you can change:

1. The circumstances

2. Your focus

3. Your belief

Circumstances

My former coworker Paul had taken up jogging to lose weight and get back into shape. Things went well for the first month, but then his knees started bothering him, first during the second half of his jogs and then at various other times during the day. He was seriously considering giving up jogging.

Paul asked for my advice. When I probed into the specifics of his routine, I discovered that he was jogging on a highly crowned road, always staying on the same side of the street. The slanted surface he was jogging on created a misalignment that placed a strain on his knees. After I had him switch his running route to include more flat roads and both sides of the street, his knee pain gradually disappeared and he was able to continue with his jogging. This is an example of how changing circumstance, in this case his running route, was able to resolve the discomfort he was experiencing.

Focus

Swimming is one of my favorite activities. I enjoy the unique sensation of propelling myself through the water and having my body fully engaged from head to toe. It provides me with a feeling of both power and grace. I find the rhythmic movement and breathing almost meditative.

Despite all of this, it's a workout I used to struggle to get myself to do. Why? I just hate getting into cold water. I dreaded the first couple of minutes before I adjusted to its temperature. It was silly to let two or three minutes of discomfort keep me from the joys of my 45-minute swim, but it demonstrates how powerful our avoidance of discomfort can be.

There wasn't much I could do to change the circumstances. I can't adjust the temperature of a lake or public pool and can't dress differently (a wetsuit would cause me to be uncomfortably warm). Scheduling my swims for the warmest days of the week is about the extent of my ability to control the circumstances.

The more important change for me to make was to change my focus. Rather than think about the unpleasant start of my swim, I learned to focus on the fantastic finish. I feel better after swimming than after any other workout. Continuing to swim, year after year, has come from having learned to shift my attention away from what I don't like to what I do like.

Belief

Running in the rain was something I used to avoid. My favorite trails became a muddy mess, there was no glorious sunshine, and it felt as though the rain was beating me down. For many years I held the belief that running in the rain was unpleasant.

A travelling companion shared with me how much she loved to run in the rain. While traveling in Europe, we ran in the rain together and I got to experience it the way she did. We enjoyed the freshness in the air, the almost musical tones created by the pattering of rain on rooftops, the comfortable temperature for running, the tranquility, the feeling of being cleansed, a feeling of returning to the reckless abandon of youth, and the idea that the rain would bring growth and life. With all of the wonderful sights and experiences we shared during the trip, our run in the rain still remains one of the more memorable events. Needless to say, my belief about running in the rain was changed and rain no longer stops me from enjoying a run.

It's usually easier to solve problems by changing our circumstances than it is by changing our focus or beliefs. For this reason, start with trying to change the circumstances to eliminate or mitigate that which you dislike. The options of how we can change our activities and routines are endless, including changing our choice of activity. For more challenging problems, look to additionally making changes in the other two areas (focus and beliefs). Using a combination of the three will solve any problem imaginable.

You'll feel better once you have come up with a good solution to a challenge you face. Solving problems often generates feelings of pride. Use this positive energy to take action implementing any portion of the solution that can be done immediately.

Embrace the Joy

Remember that exercise is not something unpleasant to be endured. Done properly, the time you exercise will be when you feel best during the day, not the worst. Your body likes to be used, but not abused. If you're miserable, figure out why. Listen to your body and let it guide you to the solution. Change what's interfering with your enjoyment.

Equally as important as identifying what isn't working well is to recognize what is. Are there logistics that make things easier or better? Does it help to leave your packed gym bag by the front door the night before? Do you prefer the stair step machine in the gym closest to the television screen? Does packing a lunch make it easier to squeeze in a lunchtime workout?

Tinker with the variables to find ways to add to your enjoyment. What clothing seems to be the most comfortable? Try active wear clothing or something designed specifically for the sport. Try adding in music or friends to enhance the experience.

During your workout, pay close attention to the enjoyable aspects. Notice how energy starts to flow through your body. Feel the release of negativity and stress. Enjoy the feeling of power coming from the flow of blood and pumping muscles. Recognize the beauty to be found in your surroundings.

> "To affect the quality of the day, that is the highest of arts."
> **Henry David Thoreau**

After completing your workout, take the time to observe how you feel. If your duration and intensity were appropriate, you'll feel invigorated, yet relaxed. You should feel good, or even great, and in a better mood than when you started. Take a moment to bask in the warmth of your well-circulated body and the glow of the post-workout sense of well-being. Take some deep breaths and notice how it's as though you are drawing in life itself. Smile and thank yourself for having given your body what it needs.

If practical, take a few minutes after your workout for focused relaxation. Lie down and make yourself comfortable. Take a few deep breaths where you release the air slowly. Focus on releasing any tension in the muscles in each part of your body. Progress from head to toe spending 30 seconds to a minute relaxing your face, neck, shoulders, arms, midsection, legs, and feet. Spend a few minutes enjoying how good your body feels at this moment.

Also take note of all the aspects of the workout that were enjoyable beyond just having your body feel better. Were you able to spend some quality time with friends or family? Was there some locker room banter that made you chuckle? Did you receive praise from someone? Did you get to catch a beautiful sunrise or sunset? There are so many extras. Notice them.

It's when you take the time to truly savor all the joy within your exercise experience that you gradually transform your associations with exercise. It's this transformation of exercise from something you feel you should do to something you want to do that forms the foundation of building your desire to exercise on a regular basis.

The Moment of Truth

Unfortunately, it takes time for feeling phenomenal to become your predominant association with exercise. It also takes time before exercise happens based on force of habit. You need to be prepared that on any given day you'll engage in an internal debate about whether to do your planned workout or not. This is normal and natural, so don't assume there's something wrong with you when it happens. When you see others at the gym diligently working away, their struggles to get themselves there aren't apparent. It's easy to think you are the only one that had a tough time. If you talk to them, though, you'll find that arriving at the gym wasn't effortless for everyone. Even those who are operating from a well-established habit will admit there are days it takes some effort to get going.

> "It is in your moments of decision that your destiny is shaped."
> **Tony Robbins**

People are wonderfully creative. We can find ways to justify virtually anything we want at any time we want. Justifying not exercising is hardly a challenge. In fact, we live in a dense forest of reasons not to. It's easy to determine we are just too busy, too tired, needing to tend to someone else's needs, deserving of a break, or to find one of a hundred other reasons.

At these times, it's important to recognize that a sure path to failure is to follow an approach of exercising only when the conditions are just right and you are in the right mood. There are always reasons to skip a workout. They're easy to identify and you could make a long list each time. Exercising only when you feel like it, free of other things you could be doing, guarantees failure.

Overcoming the Excuses

We attempt to combat the reasons why we shouldn't exercise with reasons we should. This rarely works. Whenever we say we *should* do something, there is an underlying implication it's something we would rather *not* do. In the long run, "should do" items rarely stand the test of time.

The best way to overcome rationalizations for skipping a workout is to use emotions to overpower them. Ever had a second helping at dinner even though you were on a diet? Strong desire trumps rational thought. To defeat all the reasons not to exercise, you need more than just good reasons that you should. You need a strong desire to exercise. Where does this desire come from? As mentioned in the previous section, it comes from positive associations with the exercise experience. Until these develop fully, you need to be able to vividly imagine how exercise is going to make you feel better.

Close your eyes. Set aside all of the reasons not to exercise and conjure up the positive images and good feelings you'll experience from the workout. Imagine how your body feels better: energized, refreshed, and relaxed. See how pleased you are with yourself for being good to your body by giving it what it needs. Picture how the food you ate today that you shouldn't have is vaporized by the workout. See how the rest of your day is made better with the energy boost that came from exercising.

If imagining all of the positives hasn't been convincing, shift to thinking of the bad feelings you'll have if you don't. Will you feel guilty for skipping your workout or lose some self-respect? Who, beside yourself, will be disappointed? Will you feel differently when you eat, knowing you didn't burn as many calories today?

Dissect your resistance. Determine the belief that's causing you to want to skip your workout. For example, you may be saying to yourself, "This is hard; I am so out of shape." The underlying belief here may be that your workout is going to be overly taxing and unpleasant. It could be that you've been going at it with too much intensity. But remember that unless you are a competitive athlete, exercise need not cause great discomfort. Give yourself permission to go easy if that's what it takes. An easy workout is better than none, and there's a strong chance you'll go at your normal pace once you get moving.

> "Self-pity is our worst enemy and if we yield to it,
> we can never do anything wise in this world."
> **Helen Keller**

Excuses can also be generated by a simple moment of weakness. If this is the case, purge the negative thought by picturing it going through a shredder and replace it with a positive thought, such as "I'm glad I'm getting myself into great shape." Take a deep breath and smile, knowing this is ultimately the truth.

As with almost anything you do, the more you do it, the better you get at it. Getting yourself moving is no exception. In other words, pushing yourself to not miss workouts makes it easier to not miss them in the future. Negative thoughts drain your energy, while positive thoughts strengthen it. Practice generating enough positive thoughts to overthrow the negative ones.

Sluggishness

It's common for people to decide to exercise or not based on how they feel just beforehand. Swollen glands, sore throat, cough, or other clear signs of the onset of illness are, indeed, valid reasons to ease up or skip a workout. More often, though, people experience a more general state of feeling lethargic, which they use as a reason to not exercise.

Our body gives us clues to what it needs. Our body will produce hunger pains when it wants us to eat. It will yawn when it wants us to sleep. Most people mistakenly interpret that when our body feels drained, it's telling us to rest. The real message is to change our activity level; it could be to either increase or decrease it. It's easy to know which the body needs. If you are currently working hard, the message is to ease up. If you are currently at rest, the message is to get moving.

If you are basically just sitting and feeling blasé, exercise is exactly what your body needs in order to feel good again. Just as a vacation is most needed when you have the least time for it, exercise is most needed when you least feel like doing it. Low energy and a depressed state are symptoms that your body needs exercise. Have you ever noticed that lying down and resting does little to improve this state, and, in fact, it usually just makes it worse? It takes exercise to turn things around. Stress and repressed feelings are released as you exercise. Energy is produced. Typically, the worse you feel before exercise, the better you'll feel afterward. You may be surprised how often your best workouts start with you feeling crummy.

Since effort is needed to get a workout started, the more energy you have to draw from, the easier it'll be. Employ a routine you've developed that raises your energy level as soon as the debate to exercise or not begins, and experiment to see if you can find new ways to increase either that emotional or physical energy further. Become acutely aware of people or situations which create energy drains and avoid them before your exercise time.

Wait at least 10 minutes into an activity before evaluating your enjoyment. It takes this long for the body to warm up and for the energy to start to flow. Making an immediate judgment would be like deciding the quality of your day by how you feel when you first get up in the morning. Having to drag yourself out of bed and stumble toward the bathroom doesn't mean you'll have a terrible day. It's natural to need to stoke the fire a bit to get things burning.

If you've been on the move for more than 10 minutes and you aren't starting to feel good, it's time to figure out why. Start assessing to pinpoint the problem. Is there something specific you don't like about the activity? Are you pushing too hard? What's your heart rate? Are you too hot or cold? Is something hurting? Exercise is to be enjoyed, so adjust as needed to make that happen.

Rules

We all know what rules are. They are those things that can get us into trouble when we don't obey them. Our lives are full of them and they come from many sources. The government, society, and employers all have rules for us to follow and we also have our own set of personal rules that have been evolving since childhood.

Rules create structure, which allows things to operate in a predictable fashion. Many dislike the idea of rules, because they serve to limit and control behavior, but the world would be total chaos without them. Imagine trying to drive your car if there were no speed limits and no rules of when to yield to other drivers or even which side of the road to drive on. Those who have driven in India know a bit about what this experience is like and afterward have a new appreciation of the rules of the road other countries have.

Rules serve us in many ways. They help protect us and they establish our legal rights. Like habits, rules prevent us from being overloaded with moment to moment decisions. Rules set boundaries. Frequently when we examine the worst outcomes experienced in our lives, we find they resulted from our failure to establish sufficient boundaries for either ourselves or others.

The reason there are so many rules in our lives is because they are so effective in getting results. For example, when we go on a diet, we temporarily adopt someone else's rules about what and how much to eat. The rules work and we lose weight. If we then return to our original rules about eating, which allowed us to gain weight, we will put all those pounds right back on. It's only if we change our personal rules that weight gain will be avoided in the long run.

Wednesday/Sunday Rule

The quality of your life is determined by the quality of the rules you choose to live by; get the results you want by choosing rules that serve you well. Chances are you haven't established rules when it comes to exercise. Now is the time. Adopt a personal rule that once the workweek begins, you never go past Wednesday having not yet done a workout for the week. This is to be a rule, not a guideline. This line in the sand is very powerful in maintaining your exercise habit.

Life can be hectic. When things get crazy, missing a couple of days of working out is understandable. Missing three days or more, however, means it's time to face that you aren't giving exercise enough priority. Life is not going to slow down. Exercise won't happen if it's contingent on your not being so busy.

Exercising once by Wednesday needs to be given top priority. Give up whatever you have to in order to get some type of exercise. Find a way. You may have to eat on the run, miss some tube time, or get a little less sleep, but you need to make it happen. You got to use excuses on Monday and Tuesday. There are no acceptable excuses on Wednesdays.

It doesn't have to be the workout that was planned for the day. It can be less if that's what it takes to fit it in. Just do something you can record as a workout.

Once you're at a level of doing more than one workout a week, Sundays should carry the same weight as Wednesdays in making sure you get in a second workout during the week. If it's Sunday and you have only done one workout in the past six days, it becomes another do-or-die situation. Since Wednesday you've had two weekdays and a weekend day to get it done. The time for excuses has past.

> "It does not matter how slowly you go
> as long as you do not stop."
>
> **Confucius**

Is it enough to only exercise two days a week? It's less than ideal, but rules are not designed to get the ideal behavior; rules set the outer limits of what will be tolerated. Guidelines steer us toward the ideal from within the boundaries set by rules.

Why bother struggling to do two days when it's not enough? The *2008 Physical Activity Guidelines for Americans* report is clear that any amount of physical activity is beneficial. Exercise is not an all or nothing proposition. Two days of exercise is infinitely better than doing nothing at all. The twice-a-week level serves as a minimum baseline from which it's easy to step up to more ideal activity levels. It serves the all-important purpose of keeping you in the game.

Doing a shorter workout than originally planned is not breaking the rule. When you're struggling to get yourself to do a workout, give yourself permission to cut it short. If you do different types of activities, choose your favorite. Allow yourself to start off at an easier than normal pace and to do only half of your planned workout. The important thing is to maintain your habit and routine of doing some sort of physical activity. Again, an easy workout is far superior to none at all.

Also, you may be surprised by how often you end up deciding to do the full workout after you get yourself going, despite having given yourself permission to quit early.

Dealing with Slumps

At some point, everyone will need to deal with a lapse in his or her exercise routine. It might result from an injury, illness, family problems, travel, a new job, a new home, or some other major life change. Life doles out challenges to us all. Being able to recover from a lapse is a skill that must be developed for long-term success.

People also naturally go through cycles of ups and downs physically, mentally, and emotionally. You need to be prepared for the lows that you will eventually face. If not treated, a period of decreased motivation can spread like a cancer, killing your exercise habit. For this reason, it's important to be able to recognize a slump and know how to overcome it. Not honoring the Wednesday/Sunday rule is a good indicator of the beginning of a slump.

Be Prepared

The time to start dealing with a slump is before it even happens. The middle of a slump is not the right time to figure how to get out of it. Your motivation and energy are too low by this point to have the creativity and desire for an effective solution. The remedy needs to be developed before it's needed.

In preparation for a slump, prepare visuals to keep at your disposal that will reconnect you on an emotional level with exercise. It may be a movie clip, an excerpt from a magazine or book, a personal video, photographs, or something you have written. For me, it's footage from the Tour de France and broadcast of the Hawaii Ironman Triathlon World Championships. Ready those that will work for you, keeping in mind the more items you have that will recharge your ambition, the better.

Similarly, assemble visuals of the negative results that are likely to result from not exercising. It might be your "fat pants" or whatever bigger clothes you had to wear before you got in shape. It could be a page of statistics detailing your greater chances of ending up with lifestyle diseases like heart disease or diabetes. Have a couple cards that ask good questions, like "How do you feel since you stopped exercising?" or "Do you really want to start from scratch again?"

Solutions

Identify who in your social support group would be a good person to go to for help with a slump. Often a little encouragement is all you need. Also, others can help you to see the real issue holding you back, lurking below the surface. By giving you a new perspective on your situation, they can lead you to a new approach instead of your repeating what hasn't been working.

> "Failure is simply the opportunity to begin again, this time more intelligently."
>
> **Henry Ford**

After recognizing a slump, start by forgiving yourself for having one. Maintaining an exercise program is a highly involved task with many moving parts. Breakdowns in physical states, emotional states, and logistics are bound to happen. Let go of the bad feelings to unlock the emotional energy needed to move forward. Dwelling on failure only produces more of the same. Focus on your past successes to build confidence in your ability to ultimately break through the wall you've come up against.

Remember the BEAR acronym from Chapter 3. Belief and emotion precede action. If the desire to take action is waning, either a belief or emotional attachment needs to be fortified. Review your beliefs about why exercise is important to you. Ask yourself the following questions about exercise to help guide yourself back onto your path:

- Why did I start in the first place?

- Does this original inspiring purpose still exist?

- How has it made me feel better?

- What other good things has it brought?

- Am I proud of myself when I do it?

- How do I feel when I don't?

- Will I be happy with myself if I don't go back to it?

It takes a spark to relight a flame. If the spark that got you started in the first place has less power to help you now, find a new one. Is there an upcoming event where you'd like to look your best? Do you have a busy season on the horizon that will be made easier if you enter it with a high energy level?

Overcoming a lapse is all about dealing with the problem on an emotional level. Once you know you won't be happy without returning to your exercise goals, you switch into problem-solving mode. Use the following questions to help work through the challenge:

- What is the real problem hiding behind the excuses I have been coming up with?

- What has been the benefit of allowing this problem to rule?

- Is this benefit more valuable than all of the benefits I get from exercise?

- Is this a short-term problem that will go away on its own simply with the passage of time, or is this something that will continue unless I do something about it?

- What day and time will my comeback start?

Our fitness level can decline rapidly when we stop exercising, so be conservative in deciding how much activity you start back in with. Don't feel compelled to jump in at the same level you were at when you stopped. Ease back into it. The main objective is to reestablish the habit and get back into the rhythm of exercising.

Vacations

Vacations frequently create a slump or even the end of a person's exercise routine, because they break the exercise habit. If this happens to you, follow the suggestions above to break through the slump and rebuild your momentum. To keep this from happening in the first place, you can either continue to exercise while on vacation or schedule the first workout you'll do when you return before you ever leave. Doing both is better yet.

While you may be initially reluctant to welcome exercise into your vacation, if you give it a try you'll find that it enhances the experience. This is a time to relax, and exercise helps us release tension and, therefore, more fully relax. More and more hotels are offering fitness classes or other guided activities and any well-traveled vacation destination will offer plenty of ways to have fun while being active.

If you'd rather get your exercise while also seeing the sights, set out to explore on foot or bicycle. Walking or riding allows you to experience a place more intimately, and is often the least stressful form of transportation, as it dispenses with the need for hailing taxis, renting cars, and consulting timetables. You can find bicycles to rent through some lodging establishments, rental companies that deliver a bicycle right to your door, or stations scattered throughout some cities.

Including some physical activity in your trip will maintain your exercise habit and help you avoid a slump. As an added benefit, you'll also come home feeling better than ever.

The good news is that the longer you maintain an exercise routine, the more of the benefits you'll experience and recognize. The desire to stay fit increases proportionally to the time spent enjoying fitness. This makes overcoming lapses easier each time.

In the final chapter, we'll explore further the benefits of exercise that appear gradually over time. Some of these benefits haven't yet been mentioned and may be things you've never considered. Finding an appreciation for the fullness of all benefits to be gained from your active lifestyle, however subtle, is an important milestone on your way to becoming a long-term exerciser.

CHAPTER HIGHLIGHTS

Tracking Results
- A fitness log provides accountability and maintains focus.

Conquering Challenges
- You can learn what works from what doesn't.

Embrace the Joy
- Enjoying the exercise experience leads to wanting to do more of it.

The Moment of Truth
- You may at times need to change your focus and mindset in order to get yourself to work out.

Rules
- Rules help you get the results you want.

Dealing with Slumps
- Slumps are inevitable and best prepared for in advance.

ACTION STEPS

✔ Start using a fitness log or wearable activity-tracking device.

✔ Start a habit of taking a few moments after your workout to revel in good sensations and recount everything you enjoyed.

✔ Use emotions to overcome rationalizations to skip your workout.

✔ Establish a rule you never go past Wednesday without exercising or past Sunday without exercising a second time.

✔ Prepare a plan of attack for the next time you find yourself in a slump.

Chapter 9

Your Transformation

"It is not the strongest of species that survive,
nor the most intelligent that survives. It is the one
most adaptable to change."

Charles Darwin

Path vs. Place

You have probably heard it said that life is a journey, not a destination. Life is a series of experiences, and in the end, it only matters how much joy and fulfillment we derive from them.

"So many people spend their health gaining wealth and then
have to spend their wealth to regain their health."

A.J. Reb Materi

Most often, the deepest value of exercise is not found in tangible results, but rather in being. The quality of how we live our lives on a daily basis is more important than our achievements. Many have this backward. Achieving career success, for some, is justification for a putting off exercise.

They forgo exercise so they can spend more time at the office in order to excel and ultimately live the good life. Unfortunately, the reward for doing a good job is more work. Also, the work it takes to get to the next career level is usually the same effort it takes to stay there. Ignoring the body's need for exercise becomes a lifestyle. Neglected physical needs are dealt with using unhealthy means, such as excessive caffeine, alcohol, and couch time. The good life they have worked so hard for turns out to be a mirage because the lack of exercise eventually takes its toll in reduced health and vitality, leaving little ability to enjoy it.

Decide how you want to feel each day. Do you want to feel relaxed? Do you want to feel healthy and fit? Do you want to feel energetic? Do you want to be happy with how you look? These things are difficult to achieve without exercise. Regular exercise is a necessary ingredient to the life fully lived. Why would we want anything less?

> "Research has shown that the best way to be happy is to make each day happy."
> **Deepak Chopra**

Nowadays we spend so much time staring at a screen of one type or another. Most of our time is spent up in our heads with little connection to our surroundings. Exercise has become more important than ever as a kinesthetic experience that allows us to be more present in the moment.

The body isn't designed for long periods of idleness. Do you feel stiff and sluggish when you first wake up in the morning?

Sit or lie down without allowing yourself to move a single muscle. See how long it takes until you can't stand it any longer and just have to move at least a little. The body likes to be used. To feel good you need to keep moving.

We are driven by how things make us feel to a greater extent than we often realize. If you don't feel better after exercising, make changes until you do. Change the intensity, activities, and setting until you find the combination that leaves you feeling good when you're done. How exercise feels is under your control. It can range from heart-pounding intensity to relaxing and meditative. It's your choice each day. Experiencing the feelings you want means enjoying the activities and process, not just the outcome.

We have learned responses to certain situations. Many comfort themselves when they feel lonely, sad, depressed, stressed, or upset with unhealthy food or alcohol. Drugs and alcohol are often used to dampen the effect of stress and negative energy that have been absorbed, but this does not purge it from the body. It remains and accumulates, requiring more and more consumption to treat the problem. The overconsumption creates new problems, which develop into a downward spiral.

Imagine how much better your life would be if the ways you responded to difficulties were actually good for you. Long-term exercisers have learned that exercise is a positive way to deal with life's challenges. It releases stress, instead of just masking its presence. It won't cure all of your problems, but has been proven that it will help you to better cope with them.

Progression

We all start exercising to achieve a particular outcome, typically weight loss. Anything that provides motivation to get us started is good, but the longing for this type of eventual outcome isn't enough by itself to keep us going for long. People who never progress past seeing exercise simply as a way to look better will find their attempts to incorporate exercise short-lived. By contrast, those people who recognize all the additional ways exercise makes their lives better are able to stick with it.

The benefits of exercise continue to build over time. Some can be almost immediate: stress relief, enjoyable social engagement, or a chance to get out and enjoy nature. Many come about more slowly, among them weight loss, improved muscle tone, and lower blood pressure. Other benefits possess an even more subtle and long-term nature, such as slowing the aging process. The key is to recognize and appreciate each of the benefits as they appear. This compounding of positive experiences and outcomes will build up your commitment.

Chapter 4 touched on some of the other many benefits of exercise that may not be our primary motivators. Watch for things you might experience, such as:

- Better sleep

- Fewer headaches

- Stronger immunity

- Healthier digestion

- More energy and stamina

- Better stress management

- Increased optimism and sense of well-being

Also notice how much easier the activity level you started with eventually becomes. Recognize this as a clear sign of improved health below the surface, under your skin, within your body.

Your life provides a constant stream of obstacles and pressures that threaten your intention to exercise. Often these obstacles will join forces with one another, strengthening their power. Competing commitments may surface when you're already struggling with a low energy state. Negative self-talk may join in, and before you know it, it feels as though you're facing a club-toting ogre blocking your path to exercise.

The idea of losing weight isn't enough to defeat the ogre. It's when you connect it all together—the deep-seated awareness that exercise makes you look better and feel better, that with it your body functions better and you deal with life's challenges better—that your resolve can slay the most daunting beast. You won't surrender to defeat when the value you give exercise is reflected by the diagram on page 182:

Body
Functions
Better

Look
Better

**Value of
Exercise**

Feel
Better

Handle
Life
Better

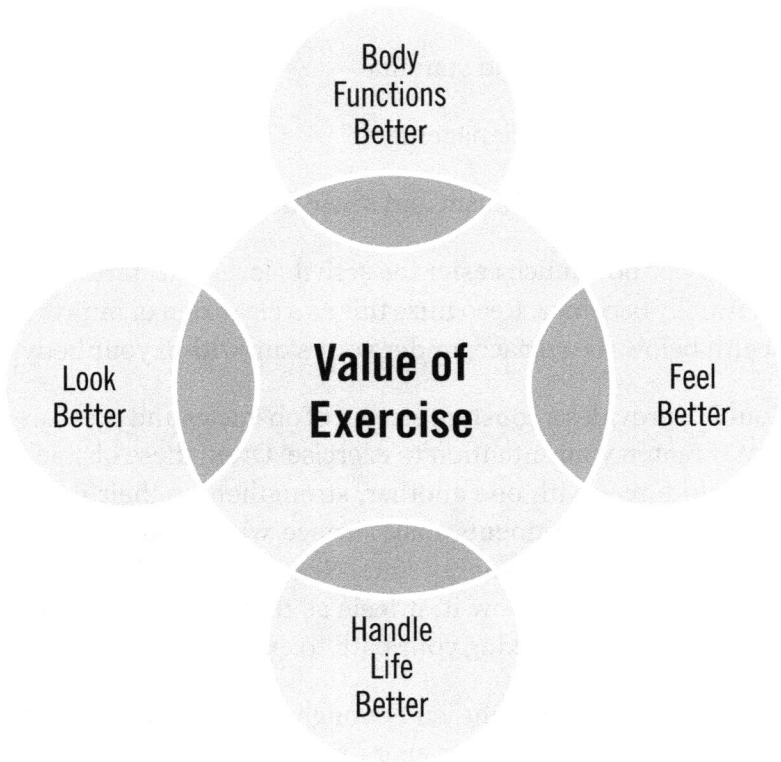

It's not enough to understand this merely conceptually. To have the necessary force and influence upon you, it must be experienced, and to experience it takes time. To stick with exercise long enough for this to happen, use the techniques you learned in previous chapters:

- Have the proper mindset

- Connect with the desired outcomes on an emotional basis

- Focus in a way that the exercise experience is enjoyed

- Create an approach that fits you and your lifestyle

- Obtain social support

- Use experience to overcome obstacles

- Use tools, like a log book and rules, to set boundaries

A lifestyle that includes fitness develops gradually over time as the components discussed in earlier chapters progressively interconnect and build upon each other. You'll stick with exercise when it becomes a form of self-expression for your core values and desires. The chart on page 184 provides an example of the evolution from first deciding to exercise to exercise being an integral part of your lifestyle.

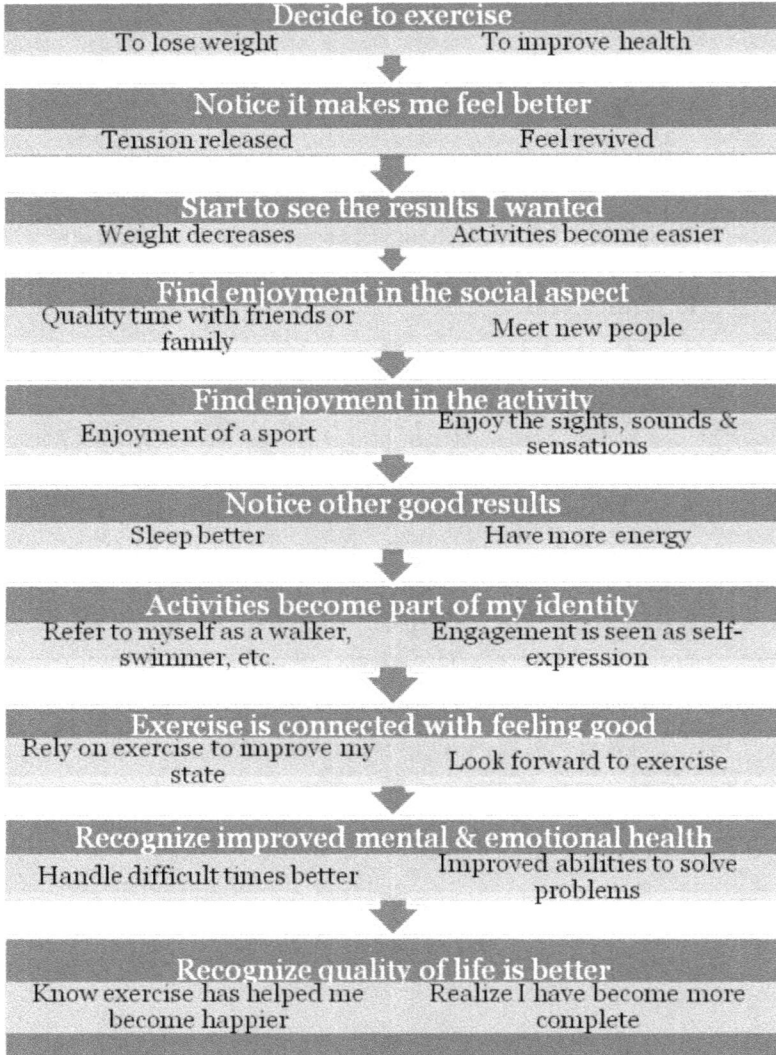

The timing, sequence, and experiences will vary among individuals, but all who have become long-term exercisers have done so through a process in which exercise progressively holds greater meaning and value.

You'll know you have crested the fitness lifestyle summit when you miss exercise when unable to do it. When you become stressed, you won't see it as a reason not to exercise; it's just the opposite. You can't wait until you have a chance to exercise, because you know this is the shortest path to feeling better.

> "Happiness is nothing more than good health and a bad memory."
> **Albert Schweitzer**

It's when you come to the point where you recognize on a deep level that exercise improves the quality of your life that you'll form a lasting attachment. When you make the connection between health and happiness, you become successful in maintaining your fitness lifestyle. Become healthier and you'll become happier. Become happier and you'll become healthier. It's in experiencing this upward spiral that you find endless commitment to exercise.

At this point, someone couldn't pay you to quit.

The Ripple Effect

Success in fitness creates success elsewhere. Countless people have gone on from achieving success in becoming fit to being more successful in other areas of their lives. It stems from much more than just the increased vitality and self-confidence that comes from exercise. It's learning to use tools like goal setting, paying attention to your energy patterns, anticipating problems, planning ahead, and solving problems when things don't go according to plan.

This is a tremendous benefit few recognize at the outset. What holds you back in one area of your life typically holds you back elsewhere. Finding the success factors in sticking with an exercise program can open the door to getting the other things out of life that have eluded you in the past. There is no more valuable skill you can develop than learning how to change yourself for the better. Behavioral change is a lifelong process. The better you become at it, the better the life you'll lead. Imagine how unstoppable you would be if you could adopt any new habit you wanted and make it stick. In light of the constantly accelerating rate of change in our world, becoming skilled at changing yourself becomes more valuable every day.

> "What you get by achieving your goals is not as important as what you become by achieving your goals."
>
> **Henry David Thoreau**

Frequently people experience an improvement in their relationships after becoming a regular exerciser. This shouldn't come as a surprise. With exercise, our disposition improves, we become better at dealing with problems and stress, our attitudes become more positive, and we're more enjoyable to be around.

Becoming a regular exerciser typically creates a positive influence on a person's diet, too. We become less dependent on food as a way to manage our state. We don't need a jelly donut to help us feel better, because we already feel good. Our interest in eating healthy food grows naturally as our self-image gradually evolves into that of a person who takes good care of his or her body. We also find ourselves craving healthier food.

Consider the confidence you'll gain from having adopted exercise as part of your lifestyle. You'll have triumphed where most others have failed. People who are fit are naturally associated with being more powerful. This is helpful in many aspects of our lives, not only because it impacts how we see ourselves, but how others see us as well. There's a certain level of respect given to those who have mastered the art of staying in shape.

I have yet to meet the long-term exerciser who regretted any of the ways exercise transformed their lives. Let exercise lead you, too, to a better life.

CHAPTER HIGHLIGHTS

Path vs. Place
- Done properly, exercise will improve how you feel on a daily basis.

Progression
- You'll see more benefits from exercise the longer you stick with it.

The Ripple Effect
- Exercise can create positive results in your life well beyond what you imagined in the beginning.

ACTION STEPS

✔ Identify how exercise fosters something you want to feel each day.

✔ If you've already started incorporating exercise into your life, determine which of the steps you've achieved in this chapter's progression chart—and start to watch for the others. If you're just beginning your journey, refer back to this chart periodically. Note your progress and keep moving toward your ultimate destination as a long-term exerciser.

✔ If you would like more information or resources, visit www.fitnesswithoutfail.com.

Selected References and Recommended Reading

Books

Brehm, Barbara A. *Successful Fitness Motivation Strategies*. Champaign: Human Kinetics Publishers, Inc., 2004.

Caldwell, Liz, and Barry Siff. *Fit and Fun For Life*. Boulder: Peak Sports Press, 2004.

Gavin, James. *Lifestyle Fitness Coaching*. Champaign: Human Kinetics Publishers, Inc., 2005.

Kimiecik, Jay. *The Intrinsic Exerciser: Discovering the Joy of Exercise*. New York: Houghton Mifflin Company, 2002.

Lencki, Tim. *Fitness One Day at a Time: Overcome the Nine Most Common Barriers to Exercise*. Lincoln: iUniverse, Inc., 2004.

Marcus, Bess H., and LeighAnn H. Forsyth. *Motivating People to Be Physically Active*. Champaign: Human Kinetics Publishers, Inc., 2009.

Menefee, Lynette A., and Daniel R. Somberg. *The Ten Hidden Barriers to Weight Loss & Exercise*. Oakland: New Harbinger Publications, Inc., 2003.

Rejeski, W. Jack, and Elizabeth A. Kenney. *Fitness Motivation: Preventing Participant Dropout*. Champaign: Human Kinetics Publishers, Inc., 1988.

Turock, Art. *Getting Physical: How to Stick with Your Exercise Program*. New York: Doubleday, 1988.

Studies / Reports

Anshel, Mark H. "Conceptualizing Applied Exercise Psychology." *The Journal of the American Board of Sports Psychology* 1-2007, Article 2.

"Interventions to Promote Physical Activity and Dietary Lifestyle Changes for Cardiovascular Risk Factor Reduction in Adults: A Scientific Statement From the American Heart Association." *Circulation* 122, no. 4 (2010): 406-441.

Rothwell, Charles, Jennifer Madans, and Jane Gentleman. *Summary Health Statistics for U.S. Adults: National Health Interview, 2012*, Vital and Health Statistics Series 10, Number 260. National Center for Health Statistics, 2014. Schoenborn, C.A., P.F. Adams, and J.A. Peregoy. *Health Behaviors of Adults: United States, 2008-2010*, Vital and Health Statistics Series 10, Number 257. National Center for Health Statistics, 2013.

U.S. Department of Health and Human Services. *2008 Physical Activity Guidelines for Americans*. 2008.

WBA Market Research. *2013 Sleep in America Poll*. National Sleep Foundation, 2013.

World Health Organization. *Global Recommendations on Physical Activity for Health.* WHO Press, 2010.

Websites

American College of Sports Medicine.
http://www.acsm.org.

American Council on Exercise.
http://www.acefitness.org.

American Heart Association. http://www.heart.org.

Centers for Disease Control and Prevention.
http://www.cdc.gov.

Healthy People 2020.
http://www.healthypeople.gov.

National Center for Health Statistics.
http://www.cdc.gov/nchs.

President's Council on Fitness, Sports & Nutrition.
http://www.fitness.gov.

World Health Organization.
http://www.who.int/en.

About the Author

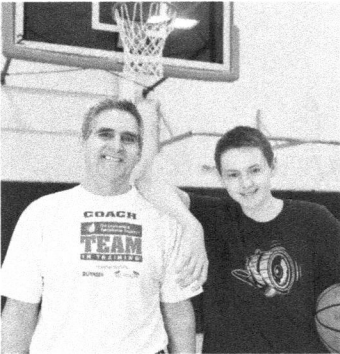

Photograph by Will Bucquoy

Bill Judson is a lifestyle fitness coach and is certified in corporate wellness and triathlon coaching. He has competed in numerous races, including such notable events as the Hawaii Ironman Triathlon World Championship and the Boston Marathon. Residing in Sonoma County, California, Bill keeps himself fit through swimming, cycling, running, hiking, kayaking, weight lifting, golfing, yoga, and playing with his son, Lance.

A lifelong passion to encourage fitness has fueled Bill's continuous study of exercise motivation. He provides engaging talks on exercise motivation for conferences, seminars, webinars, and various group meetings, and also offers consulting for wellness programs.

Additional educational information and resources may be found on his website at www.fitnesswithoutfail.com. Bill welcomes anyone to e-mail him questions, comments or stories at bjudson@fitnesswithoutfail.com.

www.ingramcontent.com/pod-product-compliance
Lightning Source LLC
Chambersburg PA
CBHW060321030426
42336CB00011B/1157